W9-CCF-267

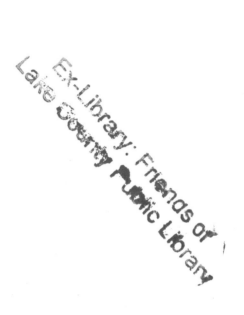

A Patient's Guide to

Dental Implants

Thomas Balshi, DDS
William Becker, DDS
Edmond Bedrossian, DDS
Peter Wöhrle, DMD

Addicus Books
Omaha, Nebraska

An Addicus Nonfiction Book

ISBN# 1-886039-65-8

Cover design by George Foster
Illustrations by Bob Hogenmiller

This book is not intended to serve as a substitute for a dental professional, nor do the authors intend to give medical advice contrary to that of an attending dental professional.

Library of Congress Cataloging-in-Publication Data

A patient's guide to dental implants / by Thomas Balshi ... [et al.].
    p. cm.
Includes bibliographical references and index.
   ISBN 1-886039-65-8
   1. Dental implants—Popular works. I. Balshi, Thomas, 1946-
RK667.I45 P38 2003
617.6'92—dc21   2002154559

Addicus Books, Inc.
P.O. Box 45327
Omaha, Nebraska 68145
www.AddicusBooks.com
Printed in the United States of America
10 9 8 7 6 5 4 3 2 1

To our wives, children, and grandchildren
who have inspired our own best smiles
through decades of faithful support as we passionately
pursued the art and science of dental medicine

Contents

Acknowledgments ix

Introduction 1

1   Why We Lose Teeth 3

2   Dental Implants: How They Work 11

3   Contemplating Dental Implant Treatment 26

4   Your Consultation 38

5   Your Dental Implant Surgery & Tooth Restoration 56

6   Caring for Your Implants 70

Resources 79

Glossary 89

Index 99

About the Authors 107

Acknowledgments

I first wish to acknowledge my first osseointegrated dental implant patient, Mr. Harry Kahn, who proved that a lifetime smile makes an incomparable difference. Additionally, I acknowledge Per-Ingvar Brånemark, for whom my practice, Prosthodontics Intermedica, was named. I also thank Dr. Ernie Mingledorff, who formed my focus on impeccable prosthodontics; and Dr. Mats Wikstrom, Mr. Ken Putney, Dr. Neil Park, and Mr. Ron Dove for decades of their genuine understanding of "partnering" to benefit patient care.

I also extend special gratitude to biomedical engineers Dr. John Brunski, Dr. Bo Rangert, and my son, Stephen F. Balshi, for ensuring that Prosthodontics Intermedica remains on the cutting edge, and to my partner Dr. Glenn Wolfinger and all the past and present staff of Prosthodontics Intermedica for delivering "A-team" dentistry.

Special thanks goes to Dr. Aureo Garcia, for carrying the torch of Prosthodontics Intermedica south of the border to Mexico City, and also to Mr. Bob Winkelman and all the dedicated staff of Fort Washington Dental Lab; they have engineered and developed many unique implant supported restorations.

I acknowledge colleagues Dr. Larry Geller, James Gentile, Dr. Sally Gupton, Dr. Charlie Goodacre, Drs. Ramon and Maria Claudia Hernandez, Dr. Ray Haggerty, Dr. Patrick Henry, Dr. Jack Crozier, Dr. Rich Cutler, Dr. Bill Viechnicki, Dr. Mike Schelkun, and Dr. Ed Woehling for sharing their knowledge and friendship. I also thank Alan Fleming and Paul Schneider, who shine light on the good things we accomplish.

Above all, I acknowledge my family, especially my wife Joanne, who has shared in every step of my professional life with unbounded loving support.

Thomas J. Balshi, D.D.S., F.A.C. P.

I would like to thank my wonderful wife Joyce, who has been unbelievably supportive of my professional activities for more than forty years. She has been my adviser and editor, always patient, always encouraging. She has spent countless hours raising two great children, running the household, editing my writing, and working in the community while I was at the computer, or lecturing, or traveling. I could not have achieved anything without her loving support. I have also been fortunate to have three outstanding mentors. It is on their shoulders that I stand. I thank Drs. John Prichard, Marshall Urist, and Clifford Ochsenbein for their willingness to teach, advise, and mentor. I thank a wonderful office support staff, three hygienists, and some of the world's greatest patients. Lastly, I thank my mother, my dad, and my partner and brother, Dr. Burton Becker. He has always supported my research and professional activities and is always there for advice and encouragement. All these people and many more have allowed me to pursue my professional interests with passion.

William Becker, D.D.S, M.S.D, O.D. (Hc)

I would like to acknowledge my mother, Nobar Bedrossian, for the gift of leadership and determination to achieve any goal I set for myself. I also thank my father, George Bedrossian, who instilled ethics, integrity, and honesty in me. These are priceless gifts for anyone to receive. My deepest gratitude to my wife, Jasmine, and my sons, Armand and Aram, for allowing me to pursue my interest and passion in the field of implant dentistry. Their patience and encouragement during the writing of this book will always be appreciated. I particularly would like to acknowledge Dr. P. I. Brånemark who has been my role model and mentor. His life-long study and unselfish dedication to research has allowed my colleagues and me to enhance the quality of life for our patients.

Edmond Bedrossian, D.D.S.

I would like to express my deep appreciation to my mentors. Dr. Paul A. Schnitman, a true clinical scholar and scholarly clinician who, as chairman of the Department of Implant Dentistry at Harvard, helped me reach my full potential. He taught me the true meaning of perseverance not by word, but by the force of a personal example. I also thank

Dr. Stephen D. Campbell, program director of postdoctoral prosthetic dentistry at Harvard, for being a role model in the pursuit of excellence.

In addition, I would like to thank all my patients. Their continuously evolving demands encourage me to seek new and better ways to make their dreams reality.

Most importantly, my deepest appreciation goes to my family. My parents taught me there are no shortcuts in the pursuit of excellence. My wonderful wife Sabine and our two children, Tess and Coco, graciously allow me to focus so much time on my passion. The smiles on the faces of my three girls make all the sacrifices worthwhile, and without them, none of this would have been possible.

Peter Wöhrle, D.M.D.

Introduction

Dental science has progressed to the point where missing teeth can be replaced with "new teeth" that are almost as good as the originals. In fact, in some ways, these new teeth called "dental implants," are even better. Unlike natural teeth, dental implants will never decay or need root canal treatments. Once they're in place, you can wear dental implants for the rest of your life.

What is your situation? Are you missing a single tooth or have you had all your teeth removed? Dental implants can be used for virtually any tooth replacement. They can replace one or more teeth, lost as a result of injury. Dental implants can be used, rather than dentures, to replace an entire set of front or back teeth that may have fallen prey to advanced periodontal disease. Implants are also effective if you are missing teeth as a result of congenital deformities of the mouth, teeth, or jaw.

We believe implants offer numerous advantages over traditional tooth replacement measures, such as bridges and dentures. The ultimate decision is, of course, yours. We hope the overview of dental implants and how they work, offered in this book, will help you make the best decisions about your dental care.

Why We Lose Teeth

A smile can speak volumes. It is part of a universal language. And probably nothing affects our smiles as much as the appearance of our teeth. We Americans spend millions of dollars a year on our teeth, all in effort to maintain or improve our appearance. We buy toothpastes with whitening agents. We buy gels "guaranteed" to brighten our smiles. In addition to these cosmetic efforts, we schedule appointments for cleanings, fillings, crowns, and root canal treatment—all with the hope of preserving our "pearly whites."

Despite all the efforts, many Americans are missing teeth and are in need of tooth replacement. According to a report on oral health from the Surgeon General, by age seventeen, more than 7 percent of the population is missing at least one permanent tooth. By age fifty, the average American is missing twelve teeth. One-third of those over sixty-five are missing all their teeth. With increasing interest, the aging population is examining options for replacing missing teeth.

Good Oral Health

The better our oral health, the less likely we are to lose teeth. What constitutes good oral health? An individual with good oral health has gums that fit snugly around the teeth. The gums are light pink and do not bleed when brushed or probed. The teeth fit together in an orderly fashion and are free of decay. The tooth's enamel is smooth and white.

A tooth has two main structures—the *clinical crown* and the *root structure.* The clinical crown is the outer, white portion, which we refer to as a "tooth." The pulp, which contains blood vessels, nerves, and arteries, is located on the inside of the tooth

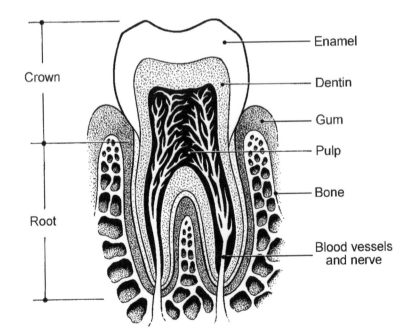

Crown

Root

Enamel

Dentin

Gum

Pulp

Bone

Blood vessels
and nerve

and extends into the root. The root structure extends into the jawbone, anchoring the tooth. The health of the root determines the long-term survival of the entire tooth. The root is like the foundation of a house—the stronger the foundation, the longer the house will last.

What Happens When Teeth Are Lost?

Aside from the cosmetics of having a missing tooth, even a small gap in your upper or lower set of teeth can create dental problems. When space is created by a missing tooth or several missing teeth, it may put stress on the remaining teeth, causing them to shift. This shifting may result in teeth that tilt and become loose. If you lose all your teeth, the gums begin to recede and the jawbone shrinks. As a result, facial tissue loses support and begins to "cave in."

Reasons for Tooth Loss

Decay

Tooth decay is, in large part, a result of not brushing and flossing our teeth adequately. When we do not properly care for our teeth, *plaque*, a sticky substance loaded with bacteria, clings to our teeth. This plaque typically forms after we have eaten sugars or starchy foods—the bacteria thrive on these foods. Accumulated plaque secretes an acid that begins to "melt away" the minerals in the tooth structure. The result is what we commonly call *cavities*; your dentist probably refers to them as *caries*.

How long does it take before the bacterial acid starts eating away at your tooth? It varies with each person; however, the acid may begin eroding the tooth's surface as soon as seventeen hours after the plaque has been allowed to collect.

Interestingly, we don't totally outgrow the tendency for tooth decay. In adults, decay often occurs around the edges of fillings or around the root structure of the tooth. If your gums recede, part of the root may be exposed. The roots are coated with *cementum*, a substance softer than enamel, making them susceptible to decay. According to the American Dental Association, the majority of people over fifty have some tooth-root decay.

Periodontal Disease

Commonly called "gum disease," *periodontal disease* is an infection of the tissues and ligaments that hold the teeth in place. These tissues are like "shock absorbers," and they stimulate bone to form next to our teeth. But the formation of bacteria and infection causes the ligaments to begin dissolving. Spaces or "pockets" form between the tooth and the gums. As bone loss occurs around the tooth, the tooth becomes loose.

Advanced periodontal disease, or *periodontitis*, is a leading cause of tooth loss among adults. Dental health professionals diagnose periodontal disease initially by examination. They'll see gums that are red and puffy and bleed easily. They confirm the diagnosis by "probing for pockets" around the gumline. A calibrated probe, similar to a very small millimeter ruler, is used to measure the depth of periodontal pockets—spaces between the gums, teeth, and bone. The pockets will have developed if the

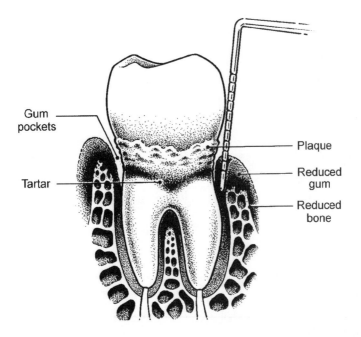

Gum
pockets

Plaque

Reduced
gum

Reduced
bone

Tartar

bone is dissolving. X-rays are also helpful in detecting the presence of periodontal disease.

Stages of Periodontal Disease

Stage I

Also known as *gingivitis*, Stage I periodontal disease is superficial inflammation of the gums, in which the gums begin to sag or pull away from the teeth. It is usually reversed with professional cleanings, followed by good hygiene—frequent brushing and flossing.

Stage II

This stage of the disease is marked by greater inflammation, swelling, and gums that bleed when touched. Pocket depths around the gums are three to five millimeters.

Stage III

A more advanced form of periodontal disease, Stage III is characterized by pocket depths of five to six millimeters. Usually more swelling is apparent, often with pus coming from the pockets, and some teeth begin to loosen in the sockets.

Stage IV

Also called "advanced periodontitis," this form of the disease involves extensive bone loss and many teeth are loose in the sockets. There is no hope for saving these teeth. They may soon fall out or will require extraction. Abscesses are frequently present.

Periodontal disease affects three out of four adults over the age of thirty-five. Although poor hygiene is a major cause of periodontal disease, other factors such as diabetes and smoking increase one's risk. For individuals whose diabetes is not controlled, circulation may be poor as a result of thickened blood vessels; consequently, cells are not nourished and do not carry away waste products efficiently. This may weaken the resistance of gum and bone tissue to infection. Smokers are five times more likely to develop gum disease. Why? Smokers have a decreased response to infection and have impaired circulation. If you are a smoker, are age forty-five or older, and have diabetes, you are twenty times more likely to develop periodontal disease.

Accidents or Trauma

Car and sporting accidents are the two major causes of broken facial bones in the United States. Understandably, many individuals lose teeth in such accidents as well. Considering all causes of accidental tooth loss, some two million teeth are lost to trauma annually. Losing even a single tooth creates more problems in the mouth than one may realize. Think of it as a "domino effect." With a gap in the teeth, the remaining teeth start shifting, pushing against other teeth. This shifting allows bacteria to accumulate more easily between the teeth, and the biting force is no longer aligned correctly. This pressure may cause bone loss, resulting in the teeth becoming loose.

In some cases a lost tooth can be reinserted; however, the tooth often becomes discolored, requires a root canal treatment, or is destroyed when the bone absorbs the root.

Congenital Anomalies

Congenital anomalies are a category of health conditions present at birth in which deviation occurs from normal growth, development, and function. The anomaly may have developed in the fetus during pregnancy or may be hereditary.

Several hereditary diseases may result in a person being born with tiny permanent teeth or no permanent teeth at all. This condition is known as *congenital anodontia,* a term referring to the complete or the partial lack of a normal number of teeth. This condition affects about 7 percent of the population. The upper lateral incisors, those next to the "front" teeth, are the most commonly absent teeth, although the lower incisors and bicuspids are also often missing.

Ectodermal dysplasia is another such congenital anomaly. It is characterized by missing teeth or by teeth that are cone- or peg-shaped. The teeth typically have defective enamel, which increases the likelihood for decay and further tooth loss. This syndrome affects males more than females and is hereditary, passed on by the mother.

Dental Implants: How They Work

For thousands of years, mankind has tried to replace missing teeth. The Etruscans are reported to have made false teeth out of ivory as early as 700 B.C. History tells us of man's ongoing efforts to create false teeth, ranging from those made with human teeth in the 1700s to the first porcelain false teeth, invented in Italy in 1837.

Moreover, archeological records show that some civilizations tried to create a crude dental implant. Egyptians and South Americans tried pounding pieces of sea shells and hand-shaped ivory into the gumline. Centuries later, in the 1800s, when implants made of human teeth failed, inventors tried gold and platinum implants. The quantum leap in oral implantology was achieved in Sweden in the early 1950s.

History of Modern Dental Implants

In 1952, in a modestly appointed laboratory in the university town of Lund, Sweden, Professor Per-Ingvar Brånemark, M.D. made a discovery by accident. A physician and researcher interested in wound healing, Dr. Brånemark was using living rabbits to study bone biology. He inserted tiny metal tubes into the rabbits' bones so that he could place a microscope to study bone tissue. The tubes were made of titanium, a light, strong, non-corrosive metal.

After several months, Brånemark attempted to remove the titanium sleeves from the rabbits' bones. Brånemark was surprised to discover that he was unable to extract them. The titanium had formed an irreversible bond with the living bone.

His curiosity aroused, Dr. Brånemark subsequently demonstrated that, under carefully controlled conditions, bone could be integrated with titanium with a very high degree of predictability. The titanium did not appear to cause inflammation in the surrounding soft tissue, nor was it rejected by the living bone. Brånemark named the process of bone bonding to titanium *osseointegration*. Before marketing his implants he spent ten years

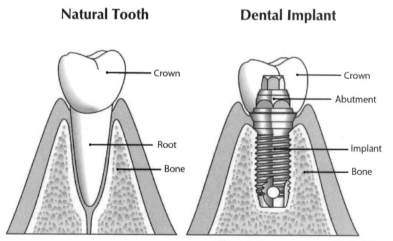

Illustration courtesy Nobel Biocare

testing them on animals and fifteen years testing them on a group of Swedish patients who had no teeth.

In 1965 the first practical application of osseointegration in dentistry was used. A man who had lost all his teeth received the first titanium dental implants. However, it was 1982 before the Food and Drug Administration gave approval for the use of titanium dental implants in the United States.

What Are Dental Implants?

Dental implants are metal posts inserted into the jawbone and serve as replacement roots for missing teeth. The replacement teeth that are later attached to the implants, look, feel, and function like natural teeth.

Implants are made of medically pure titanium, the same metal also used in the manufacture of orthopedic appliances such as hips, knees, wrists, and elbows. Thanks to the process of osseointegration, the jawbone fuses to the titanium implants, creating anchors for new, prosthetic teeth.

Dental implant-supported teeth consist of three basic components:

Implant: A titanium post or "fixture," inserted in the jawbone, which functions as an artificial root. It is often shaped like a screw.

Abutment: An extension to the implant, this cap-like device screws onto the implant and holds the artificial tooth. The abutment appears just above the gumline.

Crown: Also referred to as the "tooth."

The Implant

The average titanium implant measures one-half to three-quarters of an inch and is gently screwed or pressed into the jawbone, where it becomes the foundation for the new, prosthetic teeth. Once new bone grows around them, implants become permanent. The titanium fixtures are immovable. More than three decades of research in Sweden and the United States has recognized titanium for its biological compatibility with the human body. Studies show that the earliest patients treated with titanium osseointegrated implants continue to have good dental function.

Today, many types of implants are available for various needs of patients. There are implants for soft bone, implants that bond to bone more quickly, those that work well in very dense bone, and those for varying bone widths and heights. Implant shapes and surfaces are designed to bond quickly and predictably with the surrounding bone.

The Abutment

Also made of titanium, the abutment is a cap-like structure that is about one-third the size of the implant. The abutment is screwed into the internal thread of implant and may be positioned slightly above or even below the gumline. It provides a base on which the crown will be placed. You might think of the abutment as the "shaved down" natural tooth on which dentists cement traditional crowns.

The Crown

The crown, or prosthetic tooth, is also commonly referred to as the restoration. Crowns usually have a substructure or core that is made of metal, often gold because of its strength. In other cases, the core may be made of ceramic or zirconium, a hard, grayish-white metal that resists corrosion. The core structure is typically fused with an outer coating of porcelain, the dental material that most closely resembles the appearance of natural teeth. Crowns are custom-designed and shaded so that they look like natural teeth.

Understanding Dental Terminology

As you begin to investigate dental implants, you may come across terms that are confusing. So, let's take a moment to clarify the other common terms you will likely hear, such as "restorations," "prosthesis," "bridges," and "dentures."

Often these terms can be used interchangeably, which creates some of the confusion for those new to the topic. Perhaps this short glossary will help you navigate more smoothly.

- Restoration: This term simply refers to your teeth being restored. The words restoration and crowns are often used interchangeably. When it's time to receive your permanent crowns, you will be in the restoration phase of the process.
- Prosthesis: This term refers to your new, "man-made" teeth. They are artificial replacement teeth. "Prosthesis" could refer to a single tooth, a bridge, or a denture—all of which can be used with implants.

- Bridge: A bridge refers to several teeth, bonded together, used to fill the space where natural teeth are missing. As you're discovering, modified bridges are used with implants. A bridge is commonly referred to as a prosthesis.
- Denture: Modified dentures, also used with implants, may be referred to as a prosthesis or your prosthetic teeth. Implant-supported dentures may be removable or may be securely fastened to the implants.

Who Performs Dental Implant Surgery?

Several types of dental professionals perform dental implant surgery. Today, oral surgeons, periodontists, and prosthodontists have the most experience in implant placement.

In addition, many dentists who have received training in implant surgery provide this service. More information on the various types of dental professionals is covered in Chapter 3.

Implant Procedures

The Standard Procedure

The standard procedure for dental implant treatment takes place over a three- to six-month period. Why does it take this long? Once the implants are inserted into the jawbone, it takes several months for the bone to fuse, or osseointegrate with the titanium implants. Here's an overview of the entire three-stage process.

Stage I

In the first stage of treatment, if diseased or damaged teeth are present, they are carefully extracted with attention paid to preserving the adjacent bone. Generally, after extraction, the titanium implants are surgically inserted into the jawbone. The gums are sutured closed and the bone is allowed to fuse with the implants. So the patient won't be totally without teeth during the months the bone is attaching to the implants, he or she is usually given a temporary prosthesis to wear. The prosthesis may be a removable partial denture or a bridge that is bonded to adjacent natural teeth.

Stage II

In the second stage, three to six months later, the patient returns to the dental specialist. The patient's gums are anesthetized and a small

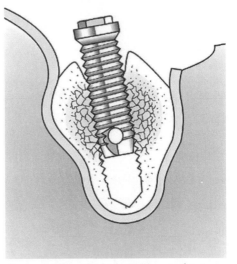

Stage I. The implant is inserted into the bone. Illustrations courtesy of Nobel Biocare.

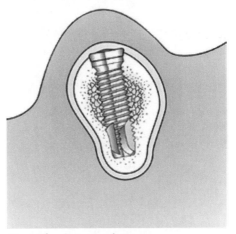

Bone fuses to implant.

17

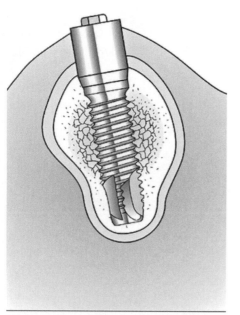

Stage II. Three to six months later, abutment is placed on the implant.

incision is made in the gum to uncover the implants. The abutments are attached to the implants. Temporary crowns are then placed on the abutments. Now the implants are capable of withstanding the pressure applied during chewing.

Stage III

Several weeks later, the dental specialist will take impressions, or imprints, of the inside of the patient's mouth, including the implant abutments, in preparation for making the permanent crowns. The impressions are sent to the dental laboratory, where a technician will make a model or cast; these casts are used to make the final implant crowns. Once the crowns are made, the patient will return to the dental office to try the crowns for fit. The dental professional will evaluate the accuracy of the fit with an x-ray. Once fitted with precision, the crowns will be affixed to the top of the implants.

This phase is referred to as *loading* the implants. The dentist makes sure the shape, color, and fit of the new teeth blend with any natural teeth.

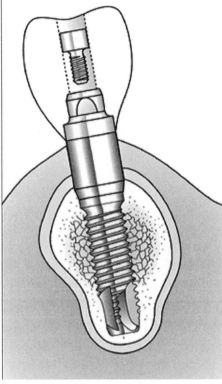

Stage III. Several weeks later the crown is placed.

The One-Stage Surgical Procedure

We have discussed the standard implant procedure involving two stages of surgery. In some instances, however, a one-stage surgical procedure can eliminate the need for a second surgery. During the one-stage operation, the dental specialist places the implants and the abutments at the same time, then he or she places the small healing caps on top of the implants. With the caps in place, the gum tissue does not grow over the implants during the months of osseointegration. With this approach, it's not necessary to have a second surgical procedure to uncover the implants.

In the one-stage procedure, the patient usually does not receive a temporary prosthesis. If he or she does receive one, it is usually a removable denture that sits loosely over the healing abutments. This denture is not stabilized or fixed to the abutments. The one-stage technique is frequently used in the back of the mouth where teeth are not visible; in these situations, temporary teeth are not really needed for cosmetic purposes.

Whether your doctor chooses to use the one-stage surgical process depends on several factors. These factors include the initial stability of the implant, the type of the implant system used, the type of temporary restoration used, and the experience and preference of the doctor. When bone grafting procedures are done at the same time as implant placement, a one-stage procedure may not advisable.

Immediately Loaded Implant Procedure

In recent years, some implant specialists have begun loading, or placing the crowns, at the same time the implants are inserted. This is referred to as an *immediately loaded implant* procedure. It is an accelerated process in which the patient makes one trip to the dentist and leaves with "teeth." No second surgery. No months of waiting. Essentially, stages one and two of the standard procedure are combined. In one procedure, the implants are inserted, the abutments are also attached to the implants, and the temporary crowns are placed.

One such immediately loaded implant procedure is the Teeth in a Day™ program. This approach is frequently used for patients who are having lower teeth replaced, since the lower jawbone is typically stronger than the upper one. The process, however, has also been used successfully in the upper jaw. Patients must also meet several criteria to be candidates for immediately loaded implants. Their clinical examinations and x-rays must show that the bone is sufficient to support the immediate placement of implants and crowns.

The implant specialist can manually determine whether the jaw can accommodate the implant (and the crowns) by gauging the tightness of the implant when it's being placed into the bone. The specialist may also elect to test the security of the implant in the bone with a machine that uses a technology called resonance frequency analysis.

Even though the entire procedure is completed in one day, it still takes several months for the bone to fuse to the titanium implants. The patient returns about three months later to receive the custom-made permanent crowns. This approach eliminates the need for the patient to wait several months between the insertion of the implants and the attachment of abutments and crowns.

Other dental implant specialists follow variations of the immediately loaded implant procedures. For example, some doctors provide a temporary fixed bridge within a few days after implant placement. Other doctors are using the immediate placement procedure in cases where a patient has lost one tooth as the result of trauma. In addition to providing an immediate cosmetic solution, the intent is to also preserve as much bone as possible by inserting the implant at the time the tooth is lost.

Replacing Teeth with Implants
Replacing a Single Tooth

If a single tooth has been cracked, broken or knocked out, an implant is often an appropriate solution. Often these patients with a missing tooth have met with some type of accident and wish to have the tooth replaced. These individuals usually have healthy

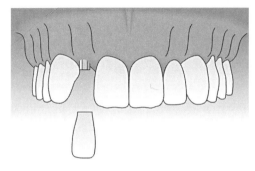

A single tooth is supported by a single implant. Illustrations courtesy of Nobel Biocare.

gums, bone, and surrounding teeth. They are usually not seeking treatment due to periodontal disease.

When a patient has a traumatized, or "injured" tooth, a restorative dentist may recommend placing the implant at the same time the traumatized tooth is removed. The single implant also allows for the restoration of the missing tooth without disturbing adjacent, natural teeth. By contrast, a conventional bridge would require shaving down the flanking teeth so the crowns, as part of the bridge, could be cemented into place.

Replacing Multiple Teeth

Generally, implants can be used to replace multiple missing teeth without disturbing adjacent healthy teeth. Whether or not to have implants depends on both x-rays of the jawbone and a clinical exam by a dental health professional. He or she will examine the health of the gum tissue and also carefully check the space created by the missing teeth to see whether it will accommodate several teeth. For example, if an individual has lost three teeth, is there adequate space to insert three implants and artificial crowns? Or have the existing teeth shifted, narrowing the space between the natural teeth?

If all criteria are met, replacing multiple missing teeth is often best accomplished with the use of an *implant bridge*, which contains one or more teeth. A bridge? Yes, a special implant bridge. If the concept of dental implants is new to you, like many individuals you may have thought a dental implant is

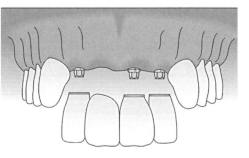

Multiple teeth are replaced by a modified bridge supported here by three implants.

a single implant screwed into place for each missing tooth. This, however, is not the case when several teeth are being replaced.

Rather, it works this way. When an implant bridge is used, a modified bridge is fabricated, similar to the traditional bridges you may have seen. However, this bridge does not attach to other natural teeth. An implant bridge is attached to the implants. The bridge holds the artificial crowns. The bridge is almost always fixed, but in special cases it may be removable. To make the bridge removable, a thin bar is placed on top of the implant abutments and the bridge clamps onto the bar. An individual may remove the teeth at will. If the bridge is fixed, there will be no bar; the bridge will be screwed or cemented onto the abutments, in which case only your dentist can remove it.

Replacing multiple teeth is usually accomplished more quickly with lower teeth than with uppers. Why? The lower jawbone is typically thicker and better suited to receiving implants. The bone in the upper arch, or upper jawbone, is capable of receiving implants; however, the bone is usually more porous and may require more weeks of healing before the abutment can be placed and temporary crowns loaded.

Replacing All Teeth

Patients who are totally *edentulous* are missing all their teeth. Depending on their oral health, these patients can receive a full set of implants by going through the standard procedure.

The approach taken is similar to the one used to replace multiple teeth. For example, rather than trying to replace all fourteen lower jaw teeth, a ten- to twelve-tooth bridge may be used with the support of only five, six, or seven implants. In the upper jaw, ten implants may be inserted to support a twelve- to fourteen-tooth bridge. Such an arrangement of implants provides teeth for chewing and is also pleasing esthetically. Similarly, a special denture may be fabricated to use with the implants.

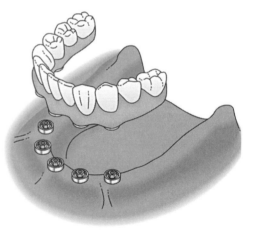

Just as the implant bridge is not a traditional bridge, an implant denture is not a traditional denture. An implant denture does not fit against the gums. Instead, the pink artificial gum of the implant denture

To replace all lower teeth, a modified bridge is placed on several implants.

rests on the abutments, which extend up through the natural gumline. As a result the special denture does not "ride" the gums. It is fixed and secure. The person wearing the implant denture has the same secure feeling with a full set of teeth as the person with one single implanted tooth.

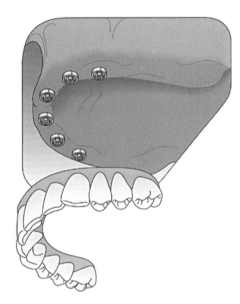

A modified bridge, placed on several implants, replaces all upper teeth.

The modified denture may be fixed or removable. The removable denture clamps to a metal bar atop the implants. The fixed denture is screwed or cemented to the implant abutment.

How Successful Are Dental Implants?

Some of the early patients have had dental implants in place for more than thirty years. Studies show success rates ranging from 90 to 97 percent for individual implants. Implants to replace the upper and lower front teeth have the highest success rates of 95 percent. These areas have greater success rates because these sections of jaws typically have the strongest bone. Upper and lower back implants have success rates of 90 to 93 percent. The bone in upper and lower back jaw is usually not as strong.

3

Contemplating Dental Implant Treatment

Are you anticipating tooth replacement? Perhaps you are missing teeth now or plan to have teeth extracted. Whichever the case, you are not alone. According to the National Institute for Dental Research, nearly 115 million Americans are missing teeth. As many as 20 million are missing all their teeth.

A growing number of Americans are exploring dental implants. In fact, the trend toward implants has tripled in the last decade. Are implants right for you? Making a choice may be easier if you better understand the differences between traditional tooth replacement and dental implant treatment.

Traditional Tooth Replacement Measures

Crowns

Often called a "cap," a traditional crown restores a tooth to its natural size, shape, and color. A crown is often used to cover a cracked or broken tooth or one that is too decayed to fill. In addition, a crown is sometimes placed for purely cosmetic reasons. Receiving a crown requires two or more visits to the dentist. During the first visit, old fillings and decay is removed, then an impression is made of the tooth so that the crown can be made to look like the original tooth. A temporary crown is placed over the tooth. During the second visit, the temporary crown is removed and the new permanent crown is cemented onto the tooth structure. The procedure helps save a tooth that would otherwise be lost.

Fixed Bridges

A *fixed bridge* is an appliance that replaces one or more missing teeth. The appliance "bridges" the gap caused by the missing tooth. It is cemented into place and can be removed only by your dental care professional. Most bridges are constructed with a "dummy crown," where the bridge is flanked by two crowns cemented onto the natural teeth on both sides of the gap. The crowns provide a solid anchor. If the natural teeth are in good condition, they may be used to anchor the bridge. Fixed bridges are a common choice among those who need tooth replacement. They are usually more attractive than dentures, and unlike dentures they have no prosthetic material covering the roof of the mouth or under the tongue. The average life of a fixed bridge is five to seven years.

Fixed bridges carry several disadvantages. The health of adjacent teeth is compromised if they are shaved down to accommodate crowns necessary for anchoring the bridge. The chance of recurrent decay around the edge of the crown or on the root also increases. The potential for gum disease increases. The anchor teeth frequently require root canal treatment.

Dentures

Full *dentures*, or "false teeth," are appliances often used by individuals who are missing all upper and/or lower teeth. Dentures are made of acrylic. There are two options for dentures. One is *immediate dentures*—the dentures are placed in the mouth immediately after the teeth are removed. *Conventional dentures*, the second option, are placed in the mouth four to eight weeks after the teeth have been removed and the gums have healed. In the case of immediate dentures, the appliance is sometimes lined with a soft material so it will sit comfortably on the gums. Conventional dentures are adjusted over a period of weeks until the fit is more comfortable.

Dentures offer several advantages. They are durable and will usually last three to five years. They improve appearance by replacing decayed or missing teeth. If you have no teeth, they make chewing easier, and aid speech; dentures are generally economical.

However, dentures also have disadvantages. Dentures may affect appearance and speech, eroding one's confidence. Gum sores may develop, making it difficult to wear the appliance. It may take several months to learn to eat with dentures, and they have only 25 percent of the chewing efficiency that natural or non-removable teeth have. The plastic roof of the denture diminishes taste. Taste is further impaired if glues are used to hold dentures in place. Even with dentures, bone loss continues, caused by the uneven pressures of the dentures "bouncing" over the gums hundreds of times a day. This process of bone shrinkage and deterioration is known as *resorption*. In the long term, this

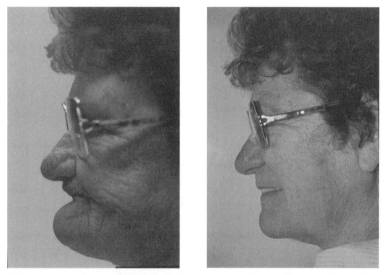

A long-term denture wearer, this woman has a "bite collapse," caused by bone shrinkage, resulting from tooth loss. At right the same woman is shown with dental implants. Photos courtesy of Quintessence Publishing Co., Inc.

may cause shrinkage and structural damage to the lower third of the face.

Partial dentures are frequently used today as an option for replacing one or several teeth. Partial dentures are made of a pink plastic base with white replacement teeth attached. Their metal framework attaches to your natural teeth with metal clasps. Partial dentures are a quick, economical solution to missing teeth, and offer essentially the same benefits as full dentures; however, they also bring similar disadvantages. Since partials clamp onto remaining, natural teeth, they may cause the natural teeth to loosen over time. Decay may develop where the clamps rest on the natural teeth.

Advantages of Dental Implants

As an alternative to traditional tooth replacement, dental implants are gaining favor around the world. The materials used to make implants are compatible with human tissue and offer greater strength and comfort than traditional dentures and bridges. Research shows the following as key reasons why the use of implants is on the rise.

- Improved appearance: Implants slow or stop bone from shrinking. Facial structure is not affected. Teeth appear natural. Bone growth is strengthened and stimulated by implants.
- Improved Comfort: Gums are not irritated or injured as they often are with moving dentures.
- Improved Speech: Implants are stable. Loose dentures may impede speech and make clicking sounds.
- Improved Eating: Chewing efficiency is similar to that of natural teeth. Ability to taste is not affected.
- Better Health: Better nutrition is possible with improved eating ability.
- Convenience: Implants are secure. You can't lose or misplace your implanted teeth.
- Reliability: Peace of mind, knowing the teeth are permanent.
- Self Esteem: Improved appearance increases confidence.

Are You a Candidate for Implants?

To undergo implant surgery, you must have reasonably good health. Some doctors say if you're healthy enough to go to the dentist to have a tooth pulled, you're probably healthy enough to have dental implants. Still, there are several factors to be considered.

Are Your Bones and Gums Healthy?

In addition to good health, one of the most important criteria for being able to have dental implants is the quality of the bone in your jawbone, where the implants will be inserted. The bone must have sufficient thickness and height to accommodate the implants. Problems with bone may arise if your jawbone has been injured in an accident, if the bone is diseased, or if you have been without teeth or worn dentures for a long time. If these problems arise, the solution is often a bone graft, which is described in detail in Chapter 4.

Also, you need to have adequate gum tissue. The dentist must check to see if the level of the gum where the tooth is missing matches that of the neighboring teeth. A check is made for any defects in the gums that may prohibit the use of an implant. The health of the teeth adjacent to the implant is important too. The presence of periodontal disease can lead to bone loss. Such loss not only affects the quality of the bone but also causes gums to pull away from the teeth. Either of these conditions would affect the esthetics of the implant.

These criteria for implants will vary, depending on whether you're replacing one tooth, several teeth, or all teeth.

What Is Your Age?

For adults there is virtually no age restriction. Although seniors often express concern that their age may prevent them from having

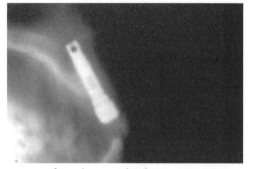

X-ray of implant with abutment

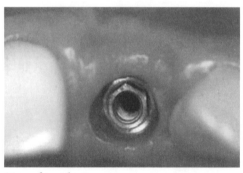

Top of implant

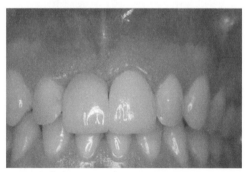

New, left front tooth

dental implants, their health is more of a determining factor than age. Patients in their 80s and 90s have permanent implant-supported teeth.

For young people, it is best that they wait to get implants until their jaws have come to maturity. This usually means age 18 for both boys and girls. However, each patient can be evaluated individually. For a child who may be missing teeth due to a congenital abnormality, an implant may be an appropriate choice.

Do You Smoke?

Just as smoking increases the risk for periodontal disease, it may also create problems for implant surgery patients. As the toxic elements from smoke enter the bloodstream, circulation may be impaired, delaying the healing process. As a result, new bone formation could be diminished and the bone may not fuse to the implant. The implant may be lost. Smoking is highly discouraged for anyone who has undergone dental implant surgery. Studies show that smokers have a higher failure rate with dental implants than nonsmokers.

What About Underlying Health Problems?

As stated earlier, if you are in reasonably good health and have adequate bone structure and gum tissue, you should be able to have dental implants. Even if you have an underlying health problem, such as heart disease or diabetes, you may have implants as long as your medical condition is well controlled. You are not at increased risk for having an implant failure.

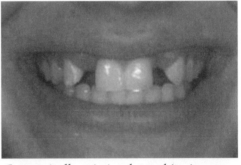

Congenitally missing lateral incisors.

What if you have osteoporosis? Many patients with osteoporosis have been successfully treated with dental implants. If you have osteoporosis, your surgeon will likely contact your physician; jointly, they will evaluate your health status and determine

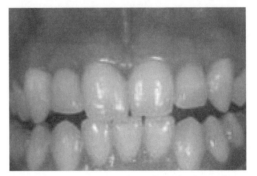

Missing incisors replaced with dental implants.

whether you should have implants. Osteoporosis by itself does not present a risk for implant placement; to date, there is also no scientific evidence that osteoporosis presents a risk for implant failure. In fact, some patients have shown increased bone deposits around their implants.

You would not be a candidate for dental implants if you have uncontrolled diabetes, are receiving chemotherapy or radiation therapy to the face or jaws, or have an untreated parathyroid disorder or blood or marrow disorder.

Finding the Right Doctor

You must choose a highly skilled, experienced doctor to perform your surgery and place your crowns. The doctor's skill is a key factor in the success of your implant treatment. If you're not sure whom to contact about dental implants, you may wish to ask your dentist. He or she may be trained in implant surgery and will treat you or will refer you to other doctors. You may also get referrals from your primary care physician as well as from family members and friends. Be cautious when responding to ads in newspapers or on TV or radio. The media does not check a doctor's qualifications before they run an ad.

Keep in mind that that you may work with one or more doctors. For example, an oral surgeon, a periodontist, or a prosthodontist may surgically insert your implants. Then another dental professional who specializes in tooth restoration may place your crowns. Or, in some cases, one doctor may perform both the surgery and place the crowns. Depending on their area of expertise, any of the following doctors may perform your implant surgery and/or placing your crowns.

Dentists

Dentists are educated and licensed to engage in all aspects of oral health. They are required to have a college degree as well as four years of training in dental school. The D.D.S. you might have noticed after your dentist's name stands for doctor of dental surgery. Some dentists hold a D.M.D. degree, meaning a doctor of dental medicine. These are equivalent degrees. All dentists must have a license to practice from the state in which they operate their practice. Dentists acquire additional training to receive one of the following titles associated with a specific dental specialty.

Prosthodontist

A prosthodontist is a dentist who has had two or more years of advanced training in cosmetic dentistry, dental implants, denture therapy and fabrication, crowns and bridges, fixed and removable partial dentures, tempro-mandibular dysfunction (TMD), facial prosthesis, and total mouth rehabilitation.

Periodontist

A periodontist is a dental specialist who diagnoses and treats the gums and supporting structures and tissues. Training takes three additional years after obtaining the D.D.S. degree. Periodontists are trained in all phases of implant surgery, bone and gum grafting, as well as non-surgical and surgical methods for treatment of periodontal disease.

Oral and Maxillofacial Surgeon

Oral and maxillofacial surgeons are dentists who have completed four to seven years of surgical training in a hospital. They specialize in surgery of the mouth, face, and jaw, including implant surgery and reconstruction of jaw defects. Oral surgeons perform bone grafting for implant patients, patients with jaw fractures, and those with facial deformities. Oral surgeons are trained to provide IV sedation and general anesthesia.

Do Dental Implants Cost More?

Dental implants cost more than traditional dentures and bridges for several reasons. A team of highly skilled professionals is involved in the process. To make a comprehensive diagnosis, dental professionals must perform several diagnostic tests. Based on their evaluation, a patient receives a highly customized treatment plan that takes into consideration overall health needs as well as the esthetic and functional requirements related to implant placement.

Some patients may require additional procedures, such as bone grafting, to ensure the long-term health of their implants. Other patients may require sleep sedation or anesthesia. In addition, implant bridges and dentures contain precious and semiprecious metals and are fused with porcelain. These must be artistically applied by experienced technicians.

Fees will also depend on the number of teeth you are having replaced and the number of implants required to support your replacement teeth. Typically there is a fee for surgical procedures and a separate fee for attaching the posts and constructing your replacement teeth. After a thorough diagnostic examination, your doctors will recommend a treatment and outline costs.

The cost for implant replacement of a single tooth is greater than the cost of a three-tooth fixed bridge. Generally, crowns and fixed bridges are expected to last about five years to seven years, while an implant should remain in your bone for the rest of your life.

In the end, the decision to have implants is a personal one. One must evaluate the cost of treatment with the physical and psychological long-range benefits that come from having secure, functional, attractive teeth.

Does Insurance Pay?

Does dental insurance pay for dental implants? Unfortunately, most insurance plans do not. Most insurance companies do not see implants as a medical necessity and will pay only for less costly restorations. Some insurance companies will pay for the special bridges or dentures used with implants but will not pay for surgical fees for the implants themselves.

4

Your Consultation

The first step for individuals considering dental implants is a consultation with a qualified professional experienced with dental implants. When making the initial appointment for evaluation, you should question the office staff regarding the length of the first visit as well as what to expect. Ask if there is any information that the doctor may need you to bring, such as your comprehensive medical and dental history forms. Having these forms completed before your first visit is a great time saver. To find out a little more about the doctor or doctors who are part of the implant team and their staff, request brochures, patient computer disks, and web sites you can review prior to your first office visit.

During your first meeting with a dental specialist, he or she will discuss with you the many different aspects of implant treatments. You can expect to talk with the specialist about the procedures that interest you, how you would benefit from them, and the surgical processes involved. If you have been referred to the specialist by another dentist for implant treatment, tell the doctor or the staff about the doctor who referred you. Be sure to pass along any information that your previous dentist provided.

Subsequent to your initial consultation, your dental professional will conduct a clinical evaluation. This evaluation may be done during your initial visit, or it may be scheduled at a later date. The evaluation may take an hour or more, depending on the complexity of your needs.

The Clinical Evaluation

Medical History

As part of collecting your medical history you will be asked questions about your dental health and general physical condition. If you have existing medical conditions, it is critical that you inform your dental specialist. For example, an illness such as diabetes can affect healing. It's also important that you list any medications you are currently taking. Dental implant surgery requires the use of various medications, so it is important to consider possible interactions with drugs you're already taking. You also need to provide a list of other physicians or dentists you've been seeing, so your implant specialist can confer with them.

Oral Exam

The doctor will examine your mouth for dental decay and periodontal disease.

Your dental specialist needs to determine how many teeth are missing, as well as the *mobility* of your teeth. Mobility, referring to whether a tooth is loose, is rated on a scale of 0 to 3. A tooth that fits snugly in the gum is rated as a 0. A very loose tooth is graded as a 3.

The doctor does an oral cancer screening, examining the tongue and all the soft tissues in the mouth. The doctor will also manually examine the patient's lymph nodes in the neck to check for any enlargements.

The entire facial symmetry is studied to determine whether facial features, including the jaws, are aligned normally. Proper alignment is important to achieving a good esthetic result.

X-rays

In addition to the standard x-rays that are done by most dentists, you may need a "panoramic x-ray." As the name implies, this x-ray gives the doctor an "all-around" or panoramic view of your jawbones and teeth, depending on the complexity of your condition. In some cases, a CT or CAT scan may be required to gather

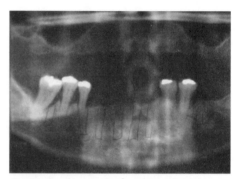

Panoramic x-ray shows patient is missing lower front teeth and all upper teeth.

additional diagnostic information. For example, a CT scan may be needed if one's teeth have been lost as the result of a traumatic injury.

Impressions

A doctor or staff member will also make *impressions* of your jaws. A tray filled with a putty-like substance will be placed in your mouth. Once hardened, this will provide a model of your teeth. This model is used for purely diagnostic purposes. It allows the doctor to determine how your teeth meet and to plan the location and number of implants needed to successfully restore your teeth. The model may also be used as a design reference for the fabrication of your new teeth.

Diagnostic Photographs

A variety of photographs are taken, including photos of your face and of your smile. These photographs document your appearance when you first visit the doctor. The photos are used as a reference for designing prosthetic replacement teeth. The doctor and the office staff may also take photos of the inside of your mouth to document your tooth and gum structure.

Shade Analysis and Selection

You and the doctor will discuss the shade or color of your natural teeth as well as the shade of any future prosthetic teeth. If you will have a combination of natural and prosthetic teeth, it's important that the shades match. Or, if you will have all new teeth, the doctor and the staff will advise you on color selection. When you receive temporary crowns, if you should find that the color of the teeth is not right for you, the color can be adjusted when the final teeth are made.

Tempro-Mandibular Joint Screening

Your doctor will also check to see if your jaws are aligned properly. Any clicking, popping, or pain in your jaw hinge could be a sign that your bite is "off," or that your jaws are not aligned correctly. These symptoms might also be caused by your chewing too heavily or grinding your teeth at night. Such habits could injure implants during the healing phase. These problems may require correction by orthodontic work, surgery, or a combination of both.

After Your Clinical Evaluation

After your clinical evaluation has been completed, you will have an opportunity to ask your doctor questions about his or her qualifications and training, as well as questions related to dental implant procedures. Understanding the answers the doctor provides is essential to feeling safe and comfortable during treatment.

Questions to Ask Your Doctor

What are your qualifications?

In addition to education and training, it is important that your dental specialist be board-certified. Board certification may vary for each specialty, but generally means that, in addition to completing dental school, a doctor has participated in an approved multi-year residency program approved by the American Dental Association. The doctor voluntarily takes a rigorous examination administered by a board which is made up of experts in the specialty.

How long have you been performing dental implant surgery or making crowns for implants?

Choose a doctor who has at least several years of experience in implant surgery and/or making crowns for implants. The skill of the doctor is a key factor in the success of your treatment. Look for a doctor who performs fifty to one hundred dental implant procedures per year.

What is your success rate?

When considering dental implant treatment it is important to know a little about statistics. Be sure to find out the doctor's statistical success rate in performing dental implants. You may have read that the overall success rate for dental implants is 95 percent; however, this statistic may have no bearing on the success rate of an individual doctor.

You should learn the doctor's success rates based on patient records. Success rates for implants vary, depending on which part of the mouth the implants are placed. For example, the success rate for implants is not as high in the upper and lower back jawbones. Implant placement and bone integration is a biologic process and is never 100 percent successful for every patient. However, an experienced surgeon should have an overall success rate of 93 percent or better.

What brand of implants do you use? How long have you been using this system? How long has the company provided implants to the dental profession?

In addition to the health of your bone and the skill of your doctor, the quality of materials used for your implants is key to the long-term success of your implants. Ask the doctor about the type of implants he or she uses and how dependable they are. Chances are you won't be familiar with the brand name, but find out why the doctor chooses that brand. How long has the doctor been using a given implant system? How dependable are they? Does the manufacturer have research that demonstrates the long-term effectiveness of the implant system? Be cautious about choosing a doctor using a new system with which he or she has little experience.

May I interview former patients?

Ask if you may speak to former patients. Personal experiences are good indicators of quality care. The dental specialist should be willing to give you names and phone numbers of patients who have agreed to be interviewed. You want to learn whether the former patient has confidence in the doctor. Was the dentist compassionate and informative, taking time to answer patient questions? Was the support staff helpful? You might ask former patients other questions such as:

- How would you describe the way the doctor dealt with you?
- Were you satisfied with the outcome of your implants?
- Did you have any problems? If so, what were they and how were they resolved?
- Did you have much pain? If so, how was it managed?
- Would you have the procedure again?
- How did implants change the quality of your life?
- What advice do you have for me, a new patient?

Where will my surgery be performed?

In some cases your surgery will be performed in the office of a dental specialist. At times the surgery is performed in hospitals or surgery centers.

Will I receive anesthesia for the surgery?

During your consultation, you should discuss your anesthesia options with your surgeon. Implant surgery may be performed with administration of local anesthetic very similar to the anesthetic given to you for routine dental fillings. However, if you would like to be completely unaware of the procedure, intravenous sedation or general anesthesia can also be administered. If you choose to have sedation, it may be administered by a dental specialist trained and certified to deliver sedation. If you choose general anesthesia, oral surgeons are trained and certified to provide this service. In some instances, a medical anesthesiologist may deliver your anesthesia.

Patients requiring sedation or general anesthesia for their procedure may need the following:

- Preoperative assessment, including health survey and possible lab tests
- Contact with the dental professional prior to the procedure to review patient's medical history
- A physical assessment on the day of the surgery
- Monitoring and administration of the anesthetic during the procedure
- Written and verbal post-operative instructions
- Telephone contact and follow-up the evening of the procedure

Patients undergoing general anesthesia should be in good health, have no evidence of chest cold, fever, or flu, and be fasting as instructed six to eight hours prior to surgery.

In my case, how long will the treatment plan take?

In standard procedures, the general rule is that implants in the lower jaw take three to four months. This means that from the time you have the implant surgery, it will be three to four months before you receive your final new teeth. The upper jaws take three to six months when following the standard treatment program.

Will I be without any teeth for months?

One of the most frequently asked questions is, "How will I look during the time my bone is healing around the implants?" Temporary replacement of teeth can be made in several ways. One method is called tooth replacement with a "flipper." This is a lightweight temporary partial denture with one or several replacement teeth attached to the partial. These can look quite good and can be removed for proper cleaning. Alternatively, a bonded bridge can be used to replace single front teeth by cementing it to the adjacent natural teeth. A bridge provides adequate esthetics, but has limited function.

How will my ability to eat be affected for the next few months while my bone is healing?

You will need to eat soft foods during the time that your bone is healing. If you are currently wearing dentures, your diet in the months ahead can be similar to your diet now; although it will need to be softer. The temporary prosthesis you will have during the healing period will be more for cosmetics than for chewing efficiency.

What about risks and complications?

Implant surgery does not carry serious risks; however, as with any surgery, complications are possible. Ask whether your dental specialist has encountered complications with other patients in the past. If so, how were the complications handled?

Infection after any type of surgery is a possible risk. Ask the doctor about safeguards to prevent infection. Surgery on the lower jaw carries a slight risk for nerve bruising, which may affect sensation of the lower lip. Such an altered sensation could resolve in weeks, or it could be permanent.

Sinus grafting in the upper jaw may pose a minor risk. During surgery, the lining of the sinus may tear. If this should occur, in most cases the injury heals without further problem.

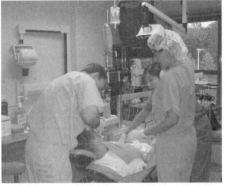

Most dental implant surgeries are performed in the office of a dental implant specialist.

When an implant is placed next to a natural tooth, it is possible that the root of the natural tooth could be affected. Such an injury may heal. Or it could result in needing a root canal treatment or in the loss of the tooth.

Is there risk of losing an implant?

A successful implant is completely anchored in bone with absolutely no mobility. A loose implant is a failed implant. Once an implant has failed or is failing, it is simply removed from its site. The site is allowed to heal for several months. During this time, bone grows to fill the space which was occupied by the implant. Once the area has healed, the specialist will evaluate the area for placement of another implant.

Implant failures are described as either early or late. Early failures usually occur between the time of implant placement and placement of the new teeth. The majority of failed implants produce minimal discomfort, infection or other symptoms. Most patients never realize that the implant has not osseointegrated.

Late implant failure, which is rare, occurs after the attachment of teeth to the implants. In some instances the amount of pressure placed during chewing exceeds the resistance, strength, or quality of your bone. If this occurs, the implants may become loose. Once the site has healed, another implant may be placed. It is important to remember that in cases where multiple implants are placed to support a bridge, failure of a single implant may not result in loss of the bridge.

How will pain be managed?

Many patients are surprised to find that they have little pain after dental implant surgery. This is especially the case if the natural teeth are already missing. Why? The ligaments which support a tooth are filled with nerve endings. Once these nerve endings are gone, the area will not be as susceptible to pain.

As with any surgery, you can expect some discomfort. During the initial surgical procedure, local anesthesia and sedatives are used to ensure that you don't feel any pain. Most patients report that they were much more comfortable following the procedure than they had anticipated. Your doctor will also give you a prescription for pain-relieving medication for use at home. Before your surgery, make sure you have received written instructions for pain management once you're home.

When can I expect to go back to work?

In almost all cases you can go back to work the following day. This is usually true for anyone having a single tooth replaced or even several. The exception would be after an operation during which all the teeth are removed and implants are placed throughout the entire jaw. Postoperative swelling may warrant staying home and keeping ice on the area to help reduce the swelling. This situation will vary from one patient to another.

If you're having more extensive surgery, such as bone grafting, you may need more time off work. Make sure you and your doctor are in agreement on the amount of time you will need to be off work so that you can plan your work schedule accordingly.

What are the costs for my treatment plan?

At the initial consultation you should receive an estimated fee, a projection of total treatment time, and a plan for fee payment. If you are treated at an implant center, the fee may include the surgery as well as restoration of the implant-supported teeth. More often, however, the surgeon's fee is separate from that of the restorative dentist or prosthodontist, and each doctor will provide an individual fee schedule. You can expect to review and sign surgical consent forms. This is standard practice throughout the United States. Make sure you read the forms completely before signing.

Can I have an MRI after getting dental implants?

Yes, you may have an MRI (magnetic resonance imaging test) after receiving implants. As you may know, the magnetic force of an MRI can create a strong pulling force on metal objects. However, titanium dental implants contain no iron. Similarly, the porcelain and gold in prosthetic crowns are not affected by the magnet.

Will dental implants set off alarms at airport security checkpoints?

No. Titanium and other dental reconstructions will not set off alarms.

Corrective Procedures

Bone Grafting

If your doctor determines that you have an insufficient amount of available jawbone for implant placement, it may still be possible for you to have implants. Procedures to build up the bone, called *bone grafting*, can be performed. Dental specialists estimate that 10 percent of patients may require such corrective procedures before they can undergo implant surgery.

Grafting is done to either widen or heighten the jawbone. The grafting helps your body regrow lost bone. The new bone growth strengthens the grafted area by forming a bridge between your existing bone and the graft. Over time, the newly formed bone will replace much of the grafted material.

One common grafting procedure involves grafting bone onto the ridge of the jawbone (the part of the bone, just under the gums, where teeth once were). This procedure is called a *ridge modification*. The gum is surgically pulled back from the jawbone, and the deformed bone is repaired. This procedure builds up the bone ridge, making it better suited for receiving implants.

Veneer Grafting

Veneer grafting refers to the process of grafting bone in order to widen the jawbone.

How is this accomplished? A piece of bone is taken from other parts of the body. In the majority of cases, bone can be taken from the lower jaw around the wisdom tooth or chin; bone from the hip can also be used. In some cases, alternative bone, such as bovine (cow) bone or chemically synthesized bone can be used to fill spaces. After four to six months of healing, the donor site will have filled with bone. It may take six to eight months for the receptor site to heal properly. When the graft matures, an implant can be placed.

The area from which the bone was borrowed will completely repair itself with new bone. The grafted site now will have proper contour for implant placement.

Onlay Grafting

Onlay grafting is used when the jawbone lacks sufficient height. The procedure builds up the bone ridge, giving it adequate height to receive an implant. This grafting helps in cases of a severely shrunken or resorbed jawbone.

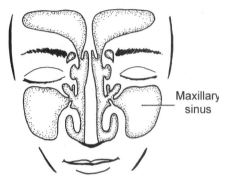

The maxillary sinuses, behind the cheeks, may require bone grafting to build up the sinus floor before an implant is inserted.

Maxillary sinus

Sinus Elevation

The upper back jaws, which are near the maxillary sinus cavities, sometimes create a problem for individuals wishing to have implants. This sinus chamber is located behind the upper cheek.

The bone in this area is generally limited and if you have a large sinus, you may have inadequate bone height for implant placement. Accordingly, your surgeon may recommend a *sinus lift* or *sinus elevation.*

A sinus lift procedure involves entering the sinus through a small incision and grafting bone into the base of the sinus cavity. This action establishes bone volume at the base of the sinus cavity, providing room for implant placement.

Grafting Gum Tissue

If you have insufficient gum tissue in an area planned to receive an implant, you may require *soft tissue grafting.* Grafting of gum tissue around a tooth or crown is occasionally needed to enhance soft tissue contours, improving the appearance. The procedure may be performed before, during, or after an implant placement. The grafts for these procedures are taken from the roof of the mouth.

This woman was missing adult teeth, the result of a birth defect.

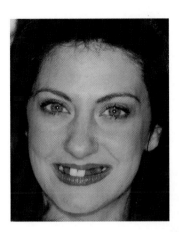

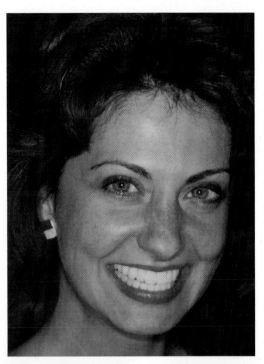

The same woman after dental implant treatment—a full implant-supported denture.

This woman had a "black tooth," resulting from nerve damage to the tooth that occurred in a childhood injury.

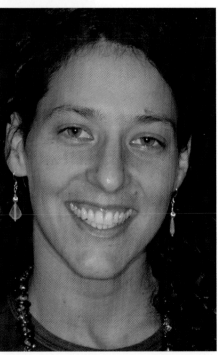

She had the "black tooth" replaced with a single dental implant. She's shown here one week after the tooth replacement.

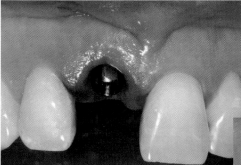

Replacing a Single Tooth

At left, front tooth is being replaced. The abutment shown is ready to receive a crown. The photo inset shows the final tooth restoration.

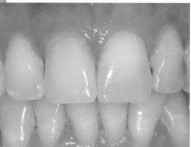

Replacing Multiple Teeth

At right, abutments are ready to receive an implant-supported bridge. Photo inset shows bridge in place.

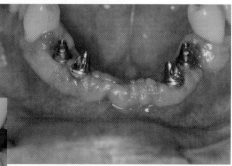

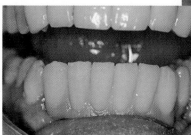

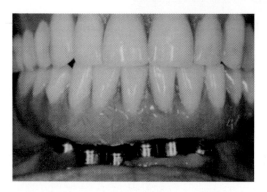

Replacing all Teeth

Implant supported dentures are shown at left. Note how the denture is placed on the abutments.

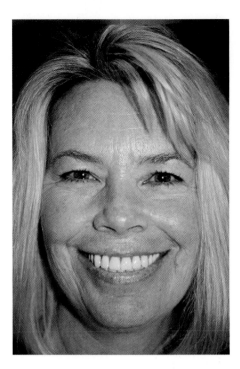

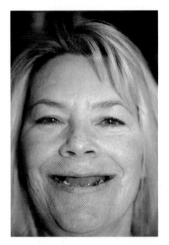

This woman lost her teeth due to periodontal disease and bone loss. Her teeth were restored with implant supported dentures.

This young man was missing many teeth, the result of ectodermal dysplasia, a birth defect. He was treated with implant-supported teeth.
Photos courtesy of Quintessence Publishing Co., Inc.

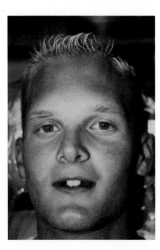

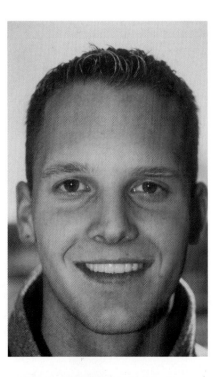

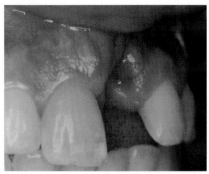

This patient lost a right front tooth and a piece of bone in an accident during adolescence.

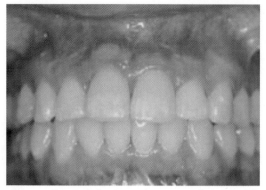

The patient underwent bone grafting to fill in the space where the bone was missing. Later, an implant was inserted in the new bone and the tooth was restored.

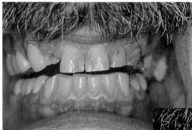

This patient had decay, old fillings, and fractured teeth.

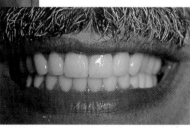

Treatment with dental implants and ceramic crowns provide a natural appearance.

This patient was missing lower, back teeth. They were restored with implant-supported crowns.

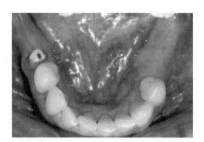

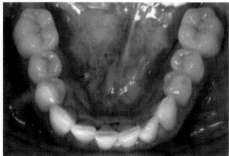

The Esthetic Zone

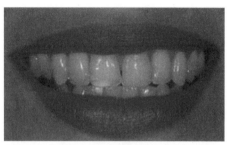

The "esthetic zone" refers to the teeth that show when one smiles. Implant-supported teeth should match one's natural esthetic zone.

Once you and your doctor have decided to move forward with dental implants, it's important to have a realistic expectation about the final outcome. During your consultation with the implant team, you will probably discuss the *esthetic zone*. This "zone" is the area of your teeth and gums that is revealed when you smile. Study of this zone is important because your newly constructed teeth need to match your natural appearance.

Some people have what's called a *low lip line* because they show only parts of their teeth while smiling. Others, with a *high lip line*, reveal all their teeth and lots of gum tissue. Since each person has a different smile, each patient has a unique esthetic zone. Any tooth replacement in the esthetic zone needs to be evaluated to judge how your smile will look when the dental work is finished.

Before you have implants, your implant specialist should be able to tell you how esthetic corrections can be made so that you have a natural-looking smile. After that, it's up to the expertise of the restorative dentist and the laboratory technician to make sure that the restoration complements your appearance.

Choosing Your Crowns

Your new teeth, or crowns, can be made from a variety of materials. Each has its advantages and disadvantages and is used accordingly. Your doctor will guide you in choosing the crowns. Virtually all patients want white porcelain crowns for their front teeth; some patients may choose gold for restoration of back teeth.

Porcelain

Most doctors recommend that porcelain materials be used for crowns that will replace a single tooth. Porcelain resembles natural teeth, and technicians can match the shade of porcelain to your natural teeth. These crowns are made by baking a porcelain veneer to either a metal or a ceramic framework. The core material provides the strength for the porcelain. The advantage of using porcelain is its esthetic outcome; the disadvantages are cost and potential fracture.

Gold

Gold restorations have been used in dentistry for decades. Gold is solid and has wear characteristics similar to natural teeth. Superior in strength to porcelain, gold does not fracture. However, for esthetic reasons, most patients don't choose all-gold crowns.

Acrylic/Composite Crowns

Acrylic composite materials are most often used for implant-supported dentures and for patients who are missing multiple teeth and have extensive gum and bone loss. The teeth for such dentures are made of a white acrylic resin veneer, which is baked onto a metal framework; pink acrylic is used to replace the missing gum and bone. These appliances are easy to maintain; however, over time the acrylic teeth wear down and will need to be replaced.

How Will Your Crowns Be Attached?

Your new teeth may be either cemented onto your implant or screwed into it. In general, single teeth or smaller restorations are cemented; larger restorations, especially all upper or lower teeth replacements, are screwed into place. There are two advantages of having a screw retained prosthesis. It's easy for the doctor to remove if lab repairs are needed, and it's easier for the doctor to examine underlying tissues.

Freestanding or Splinted Crowns

When multiple crowns are being placed, they will be placed in one of two ways. First, each crown may be separate, or freestanding. Second, they may be bonded, or "splinted," together as one piece. Deciding which method to use depends on several factors. If the implants will be under a great deal of bite force, such as that in the back of the jaw, the crowns should be splinted. Splinting them provides better distribution of pressure over the bone.

If the crowns are in the front of the mouth, where biting pressure is not as great, freestanding crowns may be used. Your doctor can best evaluate the situation and advise you.

5

Your Dental Implant Surgery
& Tooth Restoration

Y ou've completed your clinical evaluation and
made the decision to have dental implants. The
day of your surgery is approaching. You will
probably be enthusiastic about getting new teeth, but also a little
nervous about the surgery. These feelings are normal. Most patients have some anxiety about the surgery.

As previously stated in the overview of dental implants, the
three stages for a standard procedure are: the implant surgery,
abutment connection, and the final restoration, or receiving your
permanent crowns. This process can vary depending on whether
all your appointments are with one doctor at one dental center, or
whether you will be seeing more than one specialist in different
offices.

Stage 1: Implant Surgery

Preparing for Surgery

It is recommended that you wear loose clothing so that you
will be comfortable during the procedure. If you are having intra-

venous (IV) sedation or general anesthesia, plan to have a responsible adult drive you to and from the doctor's office. You are not permitted to drive a car or operate power equipment for a period of at least 24 hours following sedation or general anesthesia. You and your surgeon should have discussed any medications you take daily. In some cases, you may have been advised to discontinue a medication prior to surgery.

Just prior to your surgery, you will be given a long-acting local anesthetic, sedation or anesthesia.

Undergoing Surgery

The surgical procedure may take from one to several hours, depending on the number of implants being inserted. In most cases, you will be seated in a dental chair. It is important that the surgery be done under sterile conditions. The surgical equipment used during your procedure is sterile, and the implant is provided to your surgeon in a sterile container. The surgical assistants will have a special sterile drape which they will use to cover you. You can expect your hair to be covered and a sterile drape placed over your clothes. The implant team will also be wearing sterile gowns and gloves, as well as hats and masks.

The surgery begins with the surgeon making small incisions at the top of the gum line. The gum tissue is lifted, exposing the jawbone. The surgeon uses a series of tiny drills to make small holes in the bone.

With the holes in place, the surgeon inserts the implants. At this time the surgeon will decide whether to submerge the implant under the gum or to leave it protruding through the gum with an attached healing cap.

If the surgeon chooses to not use the healing caps, he or she will place a tiny protective cap atop each implant. These are referred to as cover screws. The gums are then closed with sutures, submerging the implant in gum tissue.

After Surgery

After your surgery, ice will be applied to the outside of your jaw to help reduce swelling. The surgical staff may take x-rays of the surgical site so the doctor can examine the placement of your implants. This will allow the doctor to evaluate the position of the implants and will be helpful in planning the next stage of treatment.

Most patients are ready to go home about thirty minutes after the surgery. Before leaving the doctor's office, you will be given a list of instructions to follow for taking medications, eating, and applying ice to the treated area. The numbness in the gums usually lasts from two to four hours.

If you're having multiple teeth replaced, you may be without teeth for the next seven to ten days. Why can't you wear a temporary denture? A denture could place pressure on the gums, causing the sutures to break open. The implants must not be disturbed during the early stages of bone healing. If they move during this healing phase, osseointegration will not occur and the implants may be lost.

In some cases the surgeon may have been able to close the incisions tightly enough to permit the patient to wear a removable denture with a soft liner. If a denture is used it is for cosmetic rather than functional or chewing purposes. No pressure should be placed on the healing incisions.

You'll be asked to return to the clinic in seven to ten days to have your sutures removed.

Recovering at Home

Once home, you will need to rest. You may be sleepy from the medications you received. If you were sedated, you should have someone stay with you until you are fully alert. While groggy, you may be prone to falling. You should not drive a car or operate any machinery immediately after your surgery.

During the first day or two at home, if you should have symptoms such as high fever, excessive bleeding, increased swelling, or excessive pain, call your doctor immediately. High fever, for example, could be a sign of infection in the bone, although infection is rare if antibiotics are being taken as directed.

Medications

After surgery, your gums and mouth may be numb for several hours. However, as the numbness of the anesthetic wears off, you may need medication for discomfort. Prior to your surgery your doctor will have given you a prescription, to be taken as you need it. The medication may be a codeine-based tablet or other type of narcotic. Some individuals find they can manage with a milder non-aspirin, over-the-counter analgesic.

You will also be given antibiotics as a precaution to minimize post-operative infections. And you may also be given a prescription mouthwash. These mouthwashes, which are referred to as *antimicrobials*, help kill bacteria. Gargle with the mouthwash as directed. Antimicrobials often have an unpleasant taste, but they help keep the tissues healthy.

Control of Minor Bleeding

Slight bleeding is not unusual after removal of teeth or following implant surgery. If you should have light bleeding, bite gently on gauze packs for thirty minutes. Remove the gauze, wait

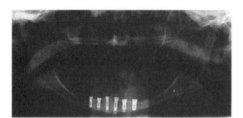

X-ray shows implants in lower jaw.

a few seconds, and see if any bleeding continues. If bleeding stops, place water-dampened gauze at the surgery site for another thirty minutes. If bleeding has stopped, no further gauze is necessary. If application of gauze does not stop bleeding on a second try, double wrap a tea bag with slightly dampened gauze and gently bite on it for forty-five minutes. Tea contains tannic acid, which can help blood clot.

Eating

Drink only liquids until the anesthetics have worn off. Proper nutrition after surgery is vital. The result of not eating correctly is fatigue, headache, dehydration, and delayed wound healing. However, you must eat only soft foods during the first several days after surgery. Avoid foods that must be broken with your teeth—hard foods such as nuts, raw vegetables, and meats that require more chewing. Many patients are comfortable with such foods as well-cooked chicken, fish, or pasta. Some individuals prefer to chop food in a blender during the first several days.

Others prefer cold foods and tepid soups. Drink at least four glasses of fluid daily.

Swelling and Bruising

After surgery, some patients experience bruising and swelling. However, the tendency to do so varies with each individual and is difficult to predict. Black and blue marks on the jaw and cheek may occur. These will fade in seven to ten days.

To control swelling, apply an ice pack to the outside of your jaw for the first twenty-four to thirty-six hours. Apply the ice pack for twenty minutes, then remove it for ten minutes to avoid injury to the skin. In place of an ice pack, a bag of frozen peas or other small vegetables may be used.

You may eat ice cream, sherbet, or any very cold liquid to aid in reduction of swelling. It's recommended you sleep on your back, with your head elevated. This helps minimize swelling by preventing lymph fluids from collecting around your jaw.

Hygiene after Implant Surgery

On the third day following surgery, gentle salt water rinses or the rinses prescribed by your doctor are permitted up to four times daily. Crushed ice or ice water may be held in your mouth. Do not vigorously rinse or spit out the ice. Either swallow the

---

Post-Surgical Guidelines

- Avoid heavy rinsing for 48 hours following surgery.
- Do not drink from a straw.
- Do not smoke until the implants are uncovered.
- Do not apply heat to the surgical area.
- Do not drink very hot beverages for 48 hours after surgery.
- Do not brush the areas adjacent to sutures.
- Do not drink carbonated beverages for 48 hours after surgery.
- Do not blow your nose hard for 48 hours, if surgery was in the upper jaw and sinuses.
- Do not skip any meals.
- Do not wear removable appliances until the sutures are removed or unless instructed to do so by your doctor.

water or let it gently run out of the mouth. Do not brush areas with sutures. Use of a water jet, set to a low pressure, is helpful. Use the water jet to clean around your natural teeth, avoiding the surgical site.

Postoperative Visits

Patients are generally asked to return to the doctor's office in seven to ten days after surgery. Depending on how you are healing, your sutures may be removed at this time; or, you may be asked to return in a few days for suture removal.

Stage II: Abutments and Crown Preparation

Three to six months after implant insertion, the implants are firmly rooted in jawbone. It's time to attach the abutments, the devices that are placed on top of the implants to hold the crowns.

Surgery to Connect Abutments

The surgeon who inserted your implants may also perform your abutment connection surgery. For this procedure, you will receive a local anesthetic to the gum area over the implants. If the healing caps have not been used, a small incision is made in the gums to expose the implants and the cover screws. Once the implants are clearly visible, the surgeon will remove the cover screws and then place the abutments into the implants. To ensure that the abutments are attached properly, the surgeon uses both manual pressure and an electronically controlled device to tighten them. The abutments are now ready to serve as the foundation for your new teeth, whether it is a bridge, denture, or even a single crown.

In some cases, the incision to expose the implants may require several sutures. This can be accomplished either before the temporary teeth are fastened to the abutments or immediately after.

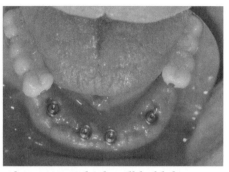

Abutments, which will hold the crowns, have been attached to the tops of this patient's implants.

After Abutment Surgery

Immediately after the abutments are connected, x-rays will be taken to assure that the abutment cylinders are properly placed. These x-rays are important to document the status of the implants and surrounding bone. These x-rays also serve as a basis for comparison of the bone structure in the years ahead.

After the abutment surgery, most patients report little discomfort. However, your gums may be tender to the touch for five to ten days. You should have very little swelling; some individuals have slight swelling of the lips or cheeks, but this is usually short in duration. In a standard procedure, you will probably be given a denture with a soft lining to wear until your final teeth are ready.

You May See Another Doctor

In some cases, the doctor who performed your surgery will also be responsible for the fabrication of your crowns. However, if your surgeon does not make your restoration he or she will refer you to another restorative dentist or prosthodontist, who will fabricate your new teeth.

Taking Impressions

After the abutments are in place, it's time to prepare for your final crowns by having impressions made of your teeth and gums. As you'll recall, you also had a set of impressions made during your clinical evaluation; however, those impressions were mostly for diagnostic purposes. This

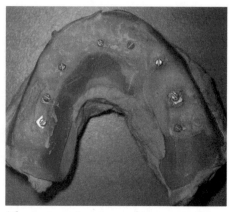

The impression is used to create the master cast on which the implant prosthesis is constructed. This impression records the precise position of the implants as they appear in the mouth.

time the dental staff will take master impressions from which your final set of teeth will be made. Taking these impressions had to wait until they could include the shape and location of the abutments.

How are the impressions made? First, a U-shaped mouth tray filled with a putty-like impression material is placed over the implants and any remaining teeth. Once the impression material has set, the tray is removed from the mouth. Now that the dental lab technicians have an exact impression of your teeth and jaws, they can pour a master stone cast. This cast precisely replicates the position of the implants in the mouth.

With the master cast made, the dental technician will make the metal framework that will hold the new teeth. The framework should be ready in about two weeks. You will be asked to schedule an appointment with your dental specialist to verify that the framework fits well. It will be screwed into place and x-rays will be taken to make sure the framework fits the abutments correctly. New computerized technology allows the frame to fit the abutments with extremely high precision.

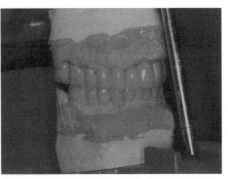

Temporary acrylic teeth fabricated in the dental lab are ready for the patient.

Hygiene after Abutment Surgery

Gentle brushing around your prosthesis and abutments is recommended if you have sutures. Cleaning between the implants may begin after the sutures are removed. You may be prescribed an antimicrobial mouthwash to use in the morning and at night.

Stage III: The Restoration

In the restoration phase, the new teeth are fabricated and fitted to the abutments. The time required by the dental lab to complete the construction of the new teeth will depend on whether a single tooth or bridge is being fabricated. This time may vary from one to two weeks or as long as six to eight weeks. Once the teeth are ready, the dental specialist will attach them to either an implant- supported bridge or denture.

Once your new custom- made teeth are attached to the abutments, they will be examined for shape, size, color, and fit.

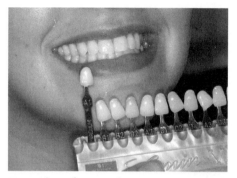

Dental professionals create a natural look with prosthetic teeth by carefully selecting the right shade of white for the crowns.

Your bite will be evaluated to make sure your upper and lower teeth are aligned. If necessary, your teeth will be adjusted.

Follow-up Visits

You'll be asked to return to the clinic in about a month, at which time the doctor will check the tightness of the prosthetic screws—the small screws that hold the teeth onto the abutment. In addition, several visits may be required to analyze and adjust your bite.

Using Night Guards

Many people clench or grind their teeth while sleeping. For those with implant-supported teeth, a night guard (mouthpiece) commonly called an occlusal guard, helps prevent fracture and wear of the teeth that may occur from grinding teeth during sleep. The guard is worn over your prosthesis. Similarly, a removable denture should not be worn during the healing phase; clenching the dentures could injure the implants.

Your doctor will probably take photographs and x-rays to use as a reference for checking for any future damage to your prosthetic (or natural) teeth from night grinding.

Post-Treatment Instructions

To ensure long-term success of your treatment, it is imperative that you keep your follow-up appointments and establish a daily hygiene maintenance routine. At your follow-up appointments, your doctor will reassess your bite, determine the stability of the prosthetic teeth, assess the condition of the gums, and evaluate bone tissue around the supporting structures. If you have an occlusal guard, be sure to take it with you to your follow-up visits.

If you detect any pain or loosening of your implant teeth, contact your dentist immediately. Eating with a loosened bridge will lead to screw fracturing and may destroy your implant-supported teeth. This may actually lead to loss of your implants.

Summary

Standard Implant Process

Before having dental implants, you will need a thorough evaluation by a dentist. The evaluation should include an oral examination, full-mouth x-rays, diagnostic casts, and photographs. This evaluation should be done less than six months prior to surgery.

Stage I Surgery

- Implants are placed in jaw
- Swelling disappears 4 to 7 days after surgery
- Sutures are removed 7 to 10 days following surgery
- Soft diet is recommended during the first 4 to 6 weeks
- Osseointegration occurs in 3 to 6 months

Stage II Surgery

- Implants are uncovered 3 to 6 months later
- Implants are checked for osseointegration
- Abutments are placed; gum tissue is sutured closed
- X-rays are taken
- Impression of mouth is done for final prosthesis
- Temporary prosthesis is made
- Sutures are removed 7 to 10 days later
- Metal framework is tested for fit

Stage III The Restoration

- Final prosthesis is completed and placed onto the implants
- Adjustments are made
- X-rays are taken

Follow-up Care

Oral hygiene maintenance is performed at three to six month intervals following placement of the final prosthesis. Regular and fastidious oral hygiene maintenance is the key to the long-term success of dental implants.

6

Caring for Your Implants

Your dental implants are wonders of biomedical engineering, but your long-term success with them depends on good oral hygiene. Keeping your prosthesis clean will prevent inflammation of the gums. And, good hygiene will prevent loss of bone around your implants and keep your prosthesis secured.

The most important times for cleaning the abutments and teeth are in the morning and in the evening. The flow of saliva slows while you are asleep. As a result, the natural cleaning action of saliva decreases, and bacterial plaque builds up.

Many areas around the dental implants need special attention to prevent dental plaque from accumulating. If you have a single tooth implant you will brush and floss normally. If you have implant dentures or a bridge, fixed or removable, the cleaning process will require a few more steps.

Cleaning Aids

In addition to traditional toothbrushes and toothpaste, the following cleaning instruments may also be helpful:

- Splayed brushes
- End-tufted brushes
- Interproximal brushes
- Electric toothbrushes
- Dental floss, multi-ply yarn, cotton ribbon
- Floss threading devices, or crochet hook
- Rubber stimulating tips
- Water irrigating devices
- Mouth rinses

Toothbrushes

A standard toothbrush is adequate to cleanse the broad surface of your prosthesis as well as the side and biting surfaces of your new teeth. If you have any natural teeth present, an American Dental Association approved, fluoridated, low abrasive toothpaste should be used.

In addition to a standard toothbrush, there are three unique brush designs that are especially helpful in removing bacterial plaque and debris from the surface of your prosthesis and the implant abutments.

Splayed Bristle Brushes

The *splayed bristle* brush, with longer bristles on each side, allows you to clean the underside of the prosthesis by rolling the bristles under the sides and bottom of the bridgework. This brush can be used in the same motions as a standard toothbrush.

End-tufted Brushes

An *end-tufted brush* is shaped like an artist's paint-brush, but with stiffer bristles. It is helpful in cleaning the tongue side of your bridgework. The end-tufted brush can access the sides of the prosthesis and the area closest to your gum tissue. If the space is available, its bristles may reach under your prosthesis and clean the outer surface of your implant abutments. The greatest advantage of the end-tufted brush is cleaning the tongue side of your lower front teeth and possibly that same area of your upper teeth.

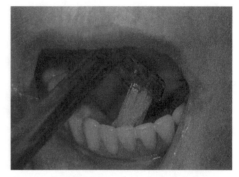

An end-tufted brush is helpful for cleaning the "back" side of your teeth.

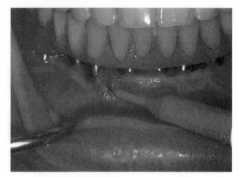

Interproximal brushes are helpful in cleaning the sides of abutment posts and the underside of the prosthesis.

Interproximal Brushes

The *interproximal brush* looks like a miniature Christmas tree. It has very soft and flexible bristles fastened to a plastic coated center wire. This brush is very useful for getting into tight places under your prosthesis and around the abutments.

Electric Toothbrushes

Electric toothbrushes are popular hygiene aids for cleaning implant-supported bridges and dentures. Why are electric toothbrushes so effective? The speed of their strokes gives them an advantage in cleaning teeth. For example, the **sonicare®**, made by Philip's Oral Healthcare, moves at 31,000 strokes per minute—about 100 times faster than we can brush manually. The high-speed bristle motion more effectively removes plaque from teeth, helping to prevent periodontal disease.

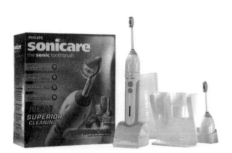

Such devices are excellent for hard to reach areas of an implant prosthesis. When using an electric toothbrush, always be careful to use gentle pressure to avoid injuring your gum tissues.

Electric toothbrushes can remove up to twice as much plaque as manual brushing. Photo courtesy of Philips Oral Heathcare, Inc.

Dental Floss and Yarn

Despite your best efforts at brushing, you may find that toothbrushes will not reach the tight spaces between your prosthesis and your gum tissue. An example of a hard-to-reach space is your upper front teeth where cosmetic demands require the prosthesis to come in direct contact with your gum tissue. In these situations, bristles from standard and special brushes may be ineffective and using dental floss ishelpful.

Various types of dental floss and soft multi-ply yarn or ribbon may be used to remove plaque from your teeth and gums. Floss threading devices that look like a crochet hook are often necessary to guide the dental floss through the narrow crevices, especially between your upper teeth and gums.

Space is often limited between the implant abutments and may preclude the use of interproximal brushes or plastic cleansing instruments, leaving dental floss as the only alternative for plaque removal.

Rubber Stimulating Tips

Some toothbrushes have rubber stimulating tips at the end. Stimulating your gums with a gentle massage using a soft rubber tip helps promote healthier gum tissue and also aids in plaque removal.

Water Irrigating Devices

Water irrigating devices in the form of a jet or spray are also quite helpful in washing away loose plaque and debris from under your implanted teeth. The strength of the pulsating jet spray should be mild so that it will not injure your gum tissue. There are many excellent irrigating devices; however, these devices will not remove all the bacterial plaque. These deposits must first be loosened by using special instruments, brushes, or floss. The irrigation flow or spray will then assist in washing away the loosened particles.

Mouth Rinses

Following the proper cleaning of your implants and artificial teeth, a thorough rinsing with an American Dental Association-approved anti-bacterial rinse, such as *chlorhexidine*, will help reduce bacterial plaque accumulations. It also helps improve the health of your gums. Scientific studies show that using these powerful mouth rinses several times a day significantly improves the health of your soft tissues, especially around your abutments by reducing bacterial plaque, which in turn lessens inflammation. Keeping your gum tissue healthy helps maintain the biologic seal around your abutments, protecting your underlying bone from bacterial invasion. Most patients who have undergone extensive implant reconstruction generally benefit from continued use of these rinses.

Cleaning Your Abutments and Prosthesis

If you have implant dentures or a bridge, the key areas to keep clean are the abutments, under the prosthesis, and the area around the gums. Doing the cleaning in front of a mirror with good lighting will be helpful. You may wish to acquire a dental mirror, a small round mirror on a handle, for checking to see if the teeth are clean.

Cleaning the Abutment Posts

Clean the sides of the abutment posts and the undersurface of the prosthesis by inserting the yarn or floss through the space next to the abutment post, around the post, and then back out the front. A floss threading device or crochet hook is helpful in passing the floss through the space and grasping it on the other side of the post to bring it forward. Then use the ribbon in a side-to-side motion to polish the back and sides from top to

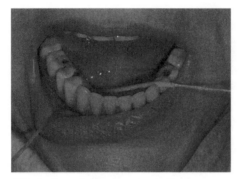

Thick dental floss or cotton yarn may be helpful in removing plaque from the sides of the abutment posts.

bottom. Adding a little toothpaste provides a very mild abrasive that will help polish the posts. Follow these procedures for each post.

Cleaning the Prosthesis

Dental floss or ribbon with a small amount of toothpaste will help you clean the underside of the prosthesis. Use the ribbon with a back-and-forth stroke, moving it from front to back. Extra-thick floss may be purchased at drugstores and may also be used for this phase of cleaning.

As mentioned, the interproximal brush will also help in the cleaning of the sides of the abutment posts and the under surface of the prosthesis. A small amount of toothpaste used with this brush may increase its ability to clean as well.

Rinsing

Always rinse your mouth thoroughly with water to remove any food particles that have been dislodged by your flossing and brushing. You may wish to complete your routine with an anti-bacterial mouthwash.

Professional Follow-up Care

Good follow-up care is a responsibility shared by you, your doctor, and your dental hygienist. The hygienist plays an important role in maintaining your implants and the surrounding tissues. He or she will show you various methods for cleaning between and beneath your implant bridges and design a custom program of oral care that you can perform at home.

At the first recall visit, your hygienist will scale and polish your abutments and your prosthesis using specially designed plastic *scalers*. These special plastic instruments help to remove deposits of plaque without scratching the surface of your abutments. Then, a special polishing paste is used to give your prosthesis a shine.

In many offices, you will see the hygienist first, and after your cleaning, the doctor will examine you. If you are having problems or if the implant bridge feels loose, notify your hygienist. He or she will evaluate the situation and make sure the doctor is aware of your concerns.

Professional Hygiene and Reevaluation Visits

Your doctor will likely recommend a follow-up treatment of oral hygiene at least four times during the first year after the completion of your first implant treatment. Then, during the second year of follow-up treatment, you will probably return every four months for professional cleaning by your dental hygienist.

Finally, after you have learned to care for your prosthesis, implants, and gum tissue, you will likely resume standard visits to your dental professional twice a year. For some patients who have an inherent tendency to accumulate bacterial deposits very quickly, more frequent professional hygiene visits may be necessary to ensure the health of the gums and bone.

Cleaning Removable Implant-Supported Teeth

If you have a screw-retained prosthesis (teeth that are held in place with small gold screws) you are probably wondering if the prosthesis should be removed at your hygiene visit. Although removal of the prosthesis often makes cleaning the abutments a much easier task for the dental hygienist, it is certainly not necessary to remove your teeth at each hygiene visit. Your implant teeth can be cleaned in your mouth, just as though they were your natural teeth.

Resources

American Dental Association
211 East Chicago Avenue
Chicago, IL 60611-2678
Phone: 800-621-8099
www.ada.org

The ADA is the professional association of dentists committed to the public's oral health, ethics, science and to professional advancement; leading a unified profession through initiatives in advocacy, education, research, and the development of standards.

The ADA and the web site offer patients and consumers oral health topics, a Find a Dentist directory, ADA Seal products, tips for teachers, children's games, and news media and video resources.

The American Academy of Cosmetic Dentistry
5401 World Dairy Drive
Madison, WI 53718

Phone: 800-543-9220

www.aacd.com

The American Academy of Cosmetic Dentistry is the largest international dental organization dedicated specifically to the art and science of cosmetic dentistry. Founded in 1984, the AACD has over 5,000 members in the United States and more than 40 countries around the world. Members of the Academy include cosmetic and reconstructive dentists, dental laboratory technicians, educators, researchers, students, hygienists, and dental assistants. The web site offers a consumer-friendly resource section.

Academy of General Dentistry

211 East Chicago Avenue, Suite 900

Chicago, IL 60611-1999

Phone: 888-342-3368

www.agd.org

Founded in 1952, the Academy of General Dentistry is a nonprofit international organization with 37,000 member dentists from the U.S., its territories, and Canada.

The Academy strives to provide the best possible patient care through the dedication of its members. In addition, it provides the patient with information to help make informed choices about personal dental care and treatments.

American Academy of Periodontology

737 North Michigan Ave., Suite 800

Chicago, IL 60611-2690

Phone: 312-787-5518

www.perio.org

The American Academy of Periodontology is a source for information about the diagnosis and treatment of periodontal disease by periodontists, experts in the diagnosis and treatment of gum disease. Their web site offers information to the public on the prevention of periodontal disease, how to protect your oral health, and locating a periodontist in your area.

American Academy of Esthetic Dentristry

401 North Michigan Avenue
Chicago, IL 60611
Phone: 312-321-5121
www.estheticacademy.org

The American Academy of Esthetic Dentistry is an organization comprised of individuals concerned with every facet of the dental profession. Members share a common interest in esthetics and excellence in the quality of patient care.

Academy of Osseointegration

85 West Algonquin Road, Suite 550
Arlington Heights, IL 60006
Phone: 800-656-7736
Fax: 847-439-1569
www.osseo.org

The Academy of Osseointegration is an international dental implant organization with a membership of over 4,200 in 70 countries. The Academy is the world's leading dental implant organization interested in bringing together individuals of different backgrounds in order to share experience and knowledge regarding implants, with the common goal of moving the field of osseointegrated implants forward.

European Academy For Osseointegration
Ms. Sarah Gold
Ms. Annie Nagem
EAO Office, 1 Wimpole Street
London, W1M8AE, UK
www.eao.org
Phone: 44-0-207-290-3948
Fax: 44-0-207-290-2989

The European Association For Osseointegration (EAO) is a nonprofit organization founded in 1991 as an international, interdisciplinary, and independent forum for all professionals interested in the art and science of osseointegration. The purposes of the Association are to foster education, clinical application, research, and improvements in the fields of reconstructive surgery and prosthetic rehabilitations.

American Academy of Maxillofacial Prosthetics
Dr. Rhonda Jacob
Anderson Cancer Center
Box 441

1515 Holcombe Boulevard
Houston, TX 77030
Phone: 713-792-6917
Fax: 713-794-4662
www.maxillofacialprosth.org

The American Academy of Maxillofacial Prosthetics (AAMP) is an association of prosthodontists who are devoted to the study and practice of methods used to increase the esthetics and function of patients with acquired congenital and developmental defects of the head and neck; and of methods used to maintain the oral health of patients exposed to radiation or cytotoxic drugs.

American Association of Oral and Maxillofacial Surgeons

9700 West Bryn Mawr Avenue
Rosemont, IL 60018-5701
Phone: 847-678-6200
www.aaoms.org

The American Association of Oral and Maxillofacial Surgeons (AAOMS) is a not-for-profit professional association serving the professional and public needs of the specialty of oral and maxillofacial surgery. Oral and maxillofacial surgeons are best noted for extracting wisdom teeth but also assist in reconstructing faces shattered by trauma, in surgically correcting misaligned jaws, and in cancer surgery of the face and neck.

American College of Prosthodontists

211 East Chicago Avenue, Suite 1000
Chicago, IL 60611
Phone: 312-573-1260
Fax: 312-573-1257
www.prosthodontics.org

The American College of Prosthodontists is the official sponsoring organization for the specialty of prosthodontics, which is one of nine recognized specialties of the American Dental Association. A prosthodontist is a dental specialist in the restoration and replacement of teeth, including crowns, bridges, inlays, complete and removable partial dentures, and dental implants; and in TMD-jaw joint problems, traumatic injuries to the mouth's structures and/or teeth, snoring disorders, and oral cancer reconstruction and continuing care.

National Foundation for Ectodermal Dysplasia

410 E. Main Street
P.O. Box 114
Mascoutah, IL 62258-0114
Phone: 618-566-2020
Fax: 618-566-4718
www.nfed.org

The Ectodermal Dysplasia syndromes (ED) are a group of genetic disorders that are identified by the absence or deficient function of at least two derivatives of the ectoderm (i.e., teeth, hair, nails, glands). The National Foundation for Ectodermal Dysplasia (NFED) is a nonprofit organization funded by the voluntary giving of individuals and organizations. NFED is the sole organization in the world providing comprehensive services to more than 3,000 families affected by ED in 50 states and more than 50 countries. The NFED is committed to improving lives by providing information on treatment and care and promoting research.

National Osteoporosis Foundation

1232 22nd Street N.W.
Washington, DC 20037-1292
Phone: 202-223-2226
www.nof.org

Osteoporosis is a disease in which bones become fragile and more likely to break. The National Osteoporosis Foundation (NOF) is the nation's leading resource for people seeking up-to-date, medically sound information on the causes, prevention, detection, and treatment of osteoporosis.

American Academy of Pediatric Dentistry

211 East Chicago Avenue, Suite 700
Chicago, IL 60611-2663
Phone: 312-337-2169
www.aapd.org

Pediatric dentists are specialists dedicated to the oral health of children and patients with special health care needs. Their web site offers parent education and answers to questions parents and children commonly ask.

American Cleft Palate-Craniofacial Association

104 South Estes Drive, Suite 204
Chapel Hill, NC 27514
Phone: 919-933-9044
800-24-CLEFT
www.cleftpalate-craniofacial.org

The American Cleft Palate-Craniofacial Association (ACPA) is an international nonprofit medical society of health care professionals who treat and/or perform research on birth defects of the head and face, including cleft lip and cleft palate. The Cleft Palate Foundation serves hundreds of families each month with free information packets to assist them in making crucial decisions about the treatment of family members with facial birth defects.

American Dental Hygienists' Association

444 North Michigan Ave., Suite 3400
Chicago, IL 60611
Phone: 312-440-8900
www.adha.org

This web site presents oral health information, including facts on proper brushing and flossing, oral cancer, periodontal disease, bad breath, nutrition, and tooth whitening systems.

National Institute of Dental and Craniofacial Research

NIDCR Public Information & Liaison Branch
45 Center Drive, MSC 6400

Bethesda, MD 20892-6400
Phone: 301-496-4261

The mission of the National Institute of Dental and Craniofacial Research (NIDCR) is to promote the general health of the American people by improving their oral, dental, and craniofacial health. Through the conduct and support of research and the training of researchers, the NIDCR aims to promote health, prevent diseases and conditions, and develop new diagnostics and therapeutics. The web site covers new research being developed as well as clinical trials.

Centers for Disease Control and Prevention
4770 Buford Highway, NE, MS F-10
Atlanta, GA 30341-3717
Phone: 770- 488-6054
CDC Voice Information System
888-CDC-FACT (888-232-3228)

This web site sponsored and updated by the Centers for Disease Control and Prevention offers oral health research that can be browsed by topic. It also offers a resource library that covers topics such as fluoride treatments, community prevention programs, infection control, and oral cancer.

International College of Prosthodontists
11276 Diamond Street
PO Box 99119
San Diego, CA 92109

Phone: 858-270-1814

www.icp-org.com

The International College of Prosthodontists (ICP) is a nonprofit public benefit corporation founded to meet the global needs for prosthodontists and their patients. The international camaraderie developed through College meetings allows the specialist to share problems and solutions with colleagues who have similar concerns and goals.

Glossary

Abrasion: Mechanical wearing away of teeth by abnormal stresses. Can result from abnormal toothbrushing habits or other abnormal stresses on the teeth.

Abutment: The connecting element between an implant and a dental crown, or prosthesis, which penetrates the gum tissue between the jawbone and the mouth.

Abutment teeth: Natural teeth used to retain and support artificial replacements for adjacent missing teeth.

Allograft: A transplant from one individual to a genetically non-identical individual.

Alloplast: Graft of a relatively inert synthetic material, usually metal, ceramic, or polymeric.

Alloys: Strong and relatively ductile, malleable metallic elements that can be polished to a high luster. Primarily made of titanium.

Alveolar bone: The bone that surrounds and supports the roots of the teeth.

Alveolar mucosa: The loosely attached mucous membrane covering the basal part of the jaw and continuing into the floor of the mouth inwardly and into the cheek vestibule outwardly.

Anatomic crown: The part of the tooth covered by enamel.

Anodontia: No teeth at all present in the jaw.

Anterior: Refers to the teeth and tissues located towards the front of the mouth.

Antimicrobial: The chemical pharmaceutical substance used to reduce bacteria in the oral cavity.

Apex: The tip of the root of a tooth or the tip of an implant.

Artificial crown: A dental replacement that restores the anatomy, function, and esthetics of a natural tooth.

Artificial root: Term used to describe dental implants.

Asepsis: Prevention from contact with microorganisms.

Attachment: A mechanical device for the fixation, retention, and stabilization of a dental prosthesis.

Bonded bridge (Maryland Bridge): Artificial replacement of one or more teeth supported by unprepared natural adjacent teeth, cemented or bonded to them.

Bridge: The artificial replacement of a missing tooth using the combination of pontics and abutment crowns.

Calculus: A calcified form of dental plaque, which must be removed with a professional cleaning.

Caps: *see* Crowns.

Caries: destruction of the enamel caused by bacteria; also known as decay.

Cavity: *see* Caries.

Cementum: Hard connective tissue covering the tooth root.

Clasp: Metal hook or clamp that binds a removable partial denture to a natural tooth.

Clinical crown: Part of the tooth that is visible above the gumline.

Complete dentures: Removable, total replacement of all teeth within one arch.

Composite defect: Clinical condition characterized by missing teeth, gum, and bone.

Congenitally: Hereditary anomaly, missing or altered from birth.

Cover screw: Device that covers and protects the top of the implant during the healing process.

Crown: Dental replacement restoring anatomy, function, and esthetics of a natural crown.

Decay: *see* Caries.

Dental implant: A modern, osseointegrated device which is placed on or within the bone associated with the oral cavity to provide support for fixed or removable prosthetics.

Dentin: The part of the tooth that is beneath enamel and cementum.

Dentures: Removable (partial or complete) set of artificial teeth.

Diastema: Space between two teeth.

Enamel: Hard calcified tissue covering dentin of the crown of tooth.

Endentulous area: Toothless area.

Endosteal implant: A smooth and/or threaded implant that is placed in the jawbone.

Esthetic zone: Visible intraoral structures defined by smile line.

Gingivitis: The initial stages of periodontal disease with inflammation of the gums.

Graft: A piece of tissue or synthetic material placed in contact with tissue to repair a defect or supplement a deficiency.

Healing cap: Device that covers and protects the top of the implant during the healing process.

High lip line: Maximum display of teeth and gums when smiling.

Immediate load: Implants that receive teeth on the day of implant placement.

Implant: Biomechanical device made from titanium, surgically inserted into the jawbone, to be used as support for artificial tooth.

Implant specialist: One who practices the art and science of implant dentistry.

Implant dentistry: The area of dentistry concerned with the diagnosis, design, and insertion of implant devices and dental restorations.

Implant denture: A denture that receives its stability and retention from a dental implant.

Implant prosthodontics: The area of implant dentistry that concerns itself with the construction and placement of fixed or removable prosthesis on any implant device.

Impression: Mold made of the teeth and soft tissues.

Mandible: Lower jawbone.

Mandibular: Pertaining to the lower jaw.

Maxilla: Upper jawbone.

One-stage procedure: Procedure that leaves part of the neck of the implant exposed above the gum immediately after implant placement.

Onlay graft: Use of solid blocks of bone to increase both the height and width of existing bony defects.

Oral surgery: That area of dentistry comprising the diagnosis and surgical treatment of diseases of the oral cavity and jaws.

Osseointegration: The biologic process of bone bonding to surface of dental implants.

Palate: The hard and soft tissues forming the roof of the mouth, which separates the oral and nasal cavities.

Partial denture or Partials: Removable replacement appliance for missing teeth, generally held in place by clasps.

Periodontal pocket: The deepened space between the gum and tooth, resulting from bone loss caused by periodontal disease.

Periodontitis: Inflammation that has spread into the underlying connective tissue and bone surrounding the teeth.

Plaque: A film of sticky material containing saliva, food particles, and bacteria that attaches to the tooth surface both above and below the gumline. When left on the tooth it can promote gum disease and tooth decay.

Pontic: Artificial replacement of an artificial tooth suspended by adjacent supporting structures, either teeth or implants.

Post: Inserted into the root of an endodontically treated tooth for the purpose of retaining a prosthetic crown.

Prosthetics: That area of dentistry that deals with problems relating to the replacement of teeth and/or jaws.

Pulp: The chamber, containing nerves and blood vessels inside the crown of a tooth.

Receptor sites: Areas in the bone or soft tissue that are prepared to receive an implant.

Resorption: Loss of bone tissue associated with the natural aging process, metabolic disturbances, or trauma.

Restoration: Any filling, inlay, crown, bridge, partial denture, or complete denture that restores or replaces lost tooth structure, teeth or oral tissues. A prosthesis.

Retread: Replacement of acrylic, composite, or denture teeth on the original gold framework of an implant supported prosthesis.

Root: The part of the tooth below the crown, normally encased in the jawbone. It is made up of dentin, includes the root canal, and is covered by cementum.

Root canal: The hollow part of the tooth's root. It runs from the tip of the root into the pulp.

Sinus lift or elevation: Bone grafting procedure within the maxillary sinus to enhance available bone volume for implant placement.

Splinting or splinted: The joining together of implants or teeth with prosthetic replacements.

Standard of care: Minimal professional standard to which dentists are accountable in their community.

Subgingiva: Below the gum line.

Glossary

Sulcus: The cuff of gum tissue around a natural tooth or an implant.

Supragingiva: Above the gum tissue.

Suspensory fibers: Ligament that joins the roots to the bone.

Torque: The force measurement used in the tightening of screw joints, such as abutments to implants.

Two-stage procedure: Submerging the implant below the gum tissue after implant placement.

Veneer graft: Use of solid blocks of bone to widen existing bone ridges.

Virgin tooth: Perfectly healthy tooth that has not received any dental treatment.

Index

A

abscesses, 8
abutment, 13, 14
    attachment, 18
    cleaning, 75, 76
    preparation, 62, 63
accidents, 9
advanced periodontitis, 8
advantages
    bridges, 27
    dental implants, 30
    dentures, 28
    partial dentures, 29
age, 31, 32
airport checkpoints, 50
American Dental Association, 6,
    42, 71, 74
anesthesia
    general, 36, 45
    local, 48
anesthesiologist, 45
antimicrobials, 59, 60
artificial replacement teeth
    see prosthesis

B

bacteria, 5, 9, 75
bacterial acid, 5, 6
bicuspids, 10
bleeding, 59
    minor, 60
blood vessels, 4
board certification, 42
bone, 4
    biology, 11, 12
    grafting, 20, 36, 49, 50, 51
    loss, 6, 9
    loss with dentures, 28
    reduced, 7
    shrinkage, 28
    sufficiency, 20, 31
Branemark, Dr. Per-Ingvar, 11–13
bridge, 15, 16, 23
    disadvantages, 27
    fixed, 23
    removable, 23
brushing 5, 71-73

C

calibrated probe, 6
candidates for
    dental implants, 30–34
caries, 5
caring for implants, 70-78
cavity, cavities, 5
    see also caries
cementum, 6
ceramic crowns, 15
chemotherapy, 34
chewing
    efficiency, 28
chlorhexidine, 75
cleaning aids, 70–75
clinical
    examination, 20, 22
clinical crown, 4
    see also tooth
clinical evaluation, 39
complications, 47, 48
congenital anodontia, 9
congenital anomalies, 9, 10
consultation, 38–55
corrective procedures, 50, 51
cosmetic dentistry, 36
cover screws, 58, 62
crown, 13, 14, 15
    acrylic, 54
    ceramic, 15
    choosing, 54, 55
    composite, 54
    conventional, 26, 27
    freestanding, 55
    gold, 54

placement, 55
porcelain, 54
preparation, 62, 63
splinted, 55
temporary, 18
CT scan, 40

D

decay, 4, 5, 6, 39
    around partial dentures, 29
    recurrent, 27
dehydration, 60
dental floss, 71, 73, 74
dental history, 38
dental implants
    advantages, 30
    brand, 43
    bridge, 23, 24
    candidates for, 30–34
    care, 70–78
    choosing crowns, 54, 55
    complications, 47, 48
    components of, 13–15
    cost, 36, 37, 49
    defined, 13
    denture, 24
    eating, 46, 58, 60, 61
    failure, 48
    failure rate, 33
    fixed denture, 25
    history, 11–13
    hygiene, 61
    immediately loaded, 20, 21
    loss, 47, 48
    modified denture, 25

Index

one-stage surgical procedure,
16-25
placement, 17
procedures, 16–25
recovery, 59–62
removable denture, 25
research, 14
restoration, 65, 66
risk factors, 47, 48
stages for standard
procedure, 16–18
standard procedure, 16–18,
68, 69
success rate, 25
surgical procedures, 56–69
terminology, 15, 16
testing, 13
treatment, 26–37
treatment plan, 46
type used, 43
dental laboratory, 18
dental professionals, 16, 34-36
dental terminology, 15, 16
dental yarn, 71, 73, 74
dentin, 4
dentist, 16, 34–36
training, 36
dentures, 15, 16
advantages, 28, 29
conventional, 28, 29
fixed, 25
immediate, 28
modified, 25
partial, 29
removable, 19, 25

risk factors of conventional,
28
risk factors of partial, 29
therapy, 36
diabetes, 33, 34
diagnostic photographs, 41
doctor
choosing, 34–36
experience, 42–44
qualifications, 42–44

E

early implant failure, 48
eating, 46, 58, 60, 61
ectodermal dysplasia, 10
edentulous, 24
electric toothbrushes, 71, 73
enamel, 4, 6
defective, 10
end-tufted brushes, 71, 72
esthetic corrections, 53
esthetic zone, 53
experience of doctor, 42-44
extraction, 17

F

facial
bones, 9
deformities, 36
tissue, 5
fatigue, 60
fever, 59
fillings, 27
finding implant specialist, 34

fixed bridges
  conventional, 27
  risk factors of conventional, 27
fixture
  see implant
flipper, 46
floss threading device, 74
flossing, 71
  lack of, 5
follow-up visits, 66, 67
  cleaning, 76–78
Food and Drug Administration, 13
freestanding crowns, 55

G

general anesthesia, 36, 45, 57
gingivitis, 7
gold crowns, 15
good hygiene, 7
grafting
  bone, 20, 49
  corrective procedures, 50, 51
  gum tissue, 52
  onlay, 51
  sinus, 47
  veneer, 51
gum disease, 6–8, 27
  see also periodontal disease
gum tissue, 57
  grafting, 52
gums, 4
  adequacy of tissue, 31
  bleeding, 8

grafting, 36
inflammation, 7, 8
receding, 5, 6
reduced, 7
sagging, 7
sores, 28
swelling, 8
tissue, 22

H

headache, 60
healing caps, 19, 57, 62
health problems, 33, 34
heart disease, 33
hereditary diseases, 9
high lip line, 53
hygiene, 5, 77, 78
  after abutment surgery, 65
  after implant surgery, 61, 62
  at home care, 70–78
hygienist, 76–78

I

immediately loaded procedure, 20, 21
implant, 13, 14
  see dental implants
  brand, 43
  bridge, 23
  complications, 47, 48
  denture, 24
  failure, 48
  loading, 18
  loss, 47, 48

placement, 17, 18
stability, 20
system, 20
type used, 43
implant-supported dentures, 16
cleaning, 78
implant team, 38
impressions, 18, 27, 40, 41
after abutment surgery, 64, 65
infection, 47, 59
inflammation, 75
insurance, 37
interproximal brushes, 71, 72
intravenous sedation, 45, 57
see also sedation

J

jawbone, 5, 13
grafting, 50, 51
heightening, 50, 51
resorption, 51
shrinkage, 51
widening, 51

L

late implant failure, 48
ligaments, 6, 48
lip line, 53
local anesthesia, 48
loose tooth rating, 39
low lip line, 53
lymph
fluids, 61
nodes, 40

M

magnetic resonance imaging
(MRI), 50
maxillary sinus, 52
medical history, 38, 39, 45
medications, 39
post-operative, 58
mobility, 39
mouth rinses, 71, 74, 75
mouthwash, 59
multiple teeth replacement,
22–24

N

National Institute for Dental
Research, 26
nerves, 4
bruising, 47
night guards, 66
Nobel Biocare, 12, 17, 22

O

occlusal guard, 66
one-stage surgical procedure,
19, 20
candidates for, 20
onlay grafting, 51
oral cancer screening, 40
oral examination, 39
oral health, 4, 5
oral surgeon, 16, 34–36
training, 36
osseointegration, 12, 13, 17, 58
after one-stage procedure, 19

osteoporosis, 33, 34

P

pain management, 48, 49
panoramic x-ray, 40
parathyroid disorder, 34
partial dentures, 29
    advantages, 28, 29
    disadvantages,
patient interviews, 44
periodontal disease, 6–8, 22, 39
    bone loss, 8
    dental aids, 73
    detection, 6
    examination, 6
    poor hygiene, 8
    risk factors, 8
    smoking, 8
    stage I, 7
    stage II, 8
    stage III, 8
    stage IV, 8
    stages, 7, 8
    treatment, 7, 36
periodontist, 16, 34–36
    training, 36
Philips sonicare®, 73
photographs
    diagnostic, 41
plaque, 5, 7, 70
pockets between tooth and
    gums, 6, 7
poor hygiene, 8
porcelain, 15
post-operative

swelling, 49, 58
visits, 62
x-ray, 58
post-treatment instructions, 67
prosthesis, 15
    see also bridge; denture; tooth
    cleaning, 75, 76
prosthetic teeth, 13, 15
prosthodontist, 16, 34–36
    training, 36
pulp, 4

Q

qualifications of doctor, 34-36,
    42

R

radiation therapy, 34
reasons for tooth loss, 5-10
recovery after surgery, 58-62
resonance frequency analysis,
    21
resorption, 28, 51
restoration, 65, 66
    see also prosthetic tooth
return to work, 49
ridge modification, 51
rinsing, 76
risk factors
    dental implants, 32, 47, 48
root
    canal treatment, 9, 27, 47
    exposure, 6
    health, 5

structure, 4
rubber stimulating tips, 71, 74

S

saliva, 70
salt water rinses, 61
scaler, 77
sedation, 36, 45
sedatives, 48
shade analysis, 18, 41, 54
shading
    see shade analysis
single tooth replacement, 21, 22
sinus
    elevation, 52
    grafting, 47
    lift, 52
    maxillary, 52
smoking, 8
    as a risk factor, 32, 33
soft tissues, 40
sonicare®, 73
splayed brushes, 71
splinted crowns, 55
stages
    of periodontal disease, 7, 8
standard implant process, 68, 69
success rate, 43
surgery
    see surgical procedures
surgical procedures, 56–69
    to connect abutments, 14, 18,
    62, 63
    to place implants, 14, 16,
    56-58

immediately loaded, 20, 21
one-stage, 19, 20
standard, 16–18
swelling, 63
gums, 8
increased, 59
post-operative, 49, 58, 61

T

tannic acid, 60
tartar, 7
taste impairment, 28
tea, 60
teeth
    abscesses, 8
    alignment, 9
    color selection, 41
    extraction, 8
    loose, 6, 8, 9
    loss, 5–10
    multiple replacement, 22–24
    periodontal disease, 6–8
    prosthetic, 13
    rating loss, 39
    replacement of all, 24, 25
    shade analysis, 41
    shading, 15
    shifting, 5, 9
    stress, 5
    tiny permanent, 9
Teeth in a Day™, 20, 21
tempro-mandibular dysfunction
    (TMD), 36, 41, 42
tempro-mandibular joint
    screening, 42

titanium, 12–14
tongue, 40
tooth
 see also clinical crown; crown
 blood vessels, 4
 bone, 4
 color selection, 41
 dentin, 4
 enamel, 4
 ligaments, 6, 48
 loose, 5, 6
 loss, 5–10
 nerves, 4
 pockets, 6
 pulp, 4
 restoration, 56–69
 shade analysis, 41
 single replacement, 21, 22
tooth loss
 due to accidents, 9
 due to periodontal disease,
  6-8
 due to trauma, 9
tooth replacement
 traditional measures, 26–29
toothbrushes, 70–75
toothpaste, 70

trauma, 9, 21, 40
treatment plan, 46
 cost, 49

V

veneer grafting, 51

W

water irrigating devices, 71, 74
work,
 returning to, 49

X

x-ray, 18
 after abutment surgery, 63
 to detect periodontal disease,
  7
 at oral exam, 40
 panoramic, 40
 post-operative, 58

Z

zirconium, 15

About the Authors

Thomas J. Balshi, **D.D.S., F.A.C.P.**, is a Diplomate of the American Board of Prosthodontists and the founder of Prosthodontics Intermedica, a resource for clinical patient care, research, and both professional and patient dental education. A graduate of Temple University and one of the U.S. pioneers in osseointegrated dental implants, Dr. Balshi trained with Professor Per Ingvar Brånemark of the Institute for Applied Biotechnology, Sweden, and 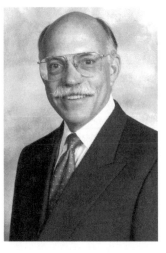 with Dr. George Zarb at the University of Toronto.

A member and past president of numerous distinguished professional organizations, Balshi was recently named to the National Academies of Practice. His life has been dedicated to advancing the science of healthy, esthetic tooth replacement, culminating in the development of Teeth in a Day,™ his trademarked process for offering patients immediate prosthetic rehabilitation in a single clinical visit.

Recognized by the U.S. Congressional Record for his scientific achievements and altruistic contributions to national healthcare, Balshi has been widely published in professional journals and has lectured internationally in such prestigious forums as the Royal College of Surgeons, the International College of Prosthodontists, and the Tissue Integration Conference in Brussels that led to the concept of Teeth in a Day.™

Balshi and his staff offer hands-on training courses for dental professionals and have produced a series of videos for patients contemplating implant treatment. The Prosthodontics Intermedica Foundation, established in 1999, offers aid to patients with severe circumstances and no financial resources. Additional information may be obtained from the Prosthodontics Intermedica web site: www.dentalimplants-USA.com

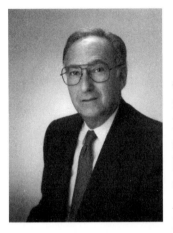

William Becker, D.D.S., **M.S.D., O.D. (hc)**, is a board-certified perio-dontist in private practice in Tucson, Arizona. He is a Diplomate of the American Board of Periodontology and has served as a board director. Becker, together with his brother, Dr. Burton Becker, has twice been awarded the prestigious Clinical Research Award from the American Academy of Periodontology. Becker is past president of the Southern Arizona Dental Society and the American Academy of Periodontology. He is a fellow of the American College of Dentists and a member of the National Academy of Practitioners. Becker is a clinical professor of periodontology at the University of Southern California School of Dentistry in Los Angeles, California. He was the Schluger Professor at the University of Washington in Seattle during 1993-94 and is presently an affiliate professor at the University of Washington. Becker has authored over eighty studies relating to periodontal therapy or dental implants and has lectured throughout the United States, Europe, the Far East and the Middle East. He is co-editor of *Clinical Implant Dentistry and Related Research.*

Becker graduated from Marquette Dental School and completed his specialty training in periodontology receiving a Master of Science Degree from Baylor College of Dentistry. In November of 1996 he received an Honorary Doctorate in Odontology from Gothenburg University in Gothenburg, Sweden

Dr. Becker may be reached by email at Branebill@ Comcast.net.

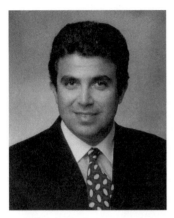

Edmond Bedrossian, **D.D.S.**, is a board-certified oral and maxillofacial surgeon in private practice in San Francisco. He is a graduate of the University of the Pacific School of Dentistry; he completed a four-year oral and maxillofacial residency training program at the Alameda Medical Center. Bedrossian is the director of the surgical implant training program at the Alameda Medical Center in Oakland, California. He also is the director of the Post-doctoral implant training program at the University of the Pacific School of Dentistry.

His academic appointments also include associate professor at the University of California at San Francisco and the University of the Pacific School of Dentistry. Bedrossian is the past president of the San Francisco Dental Society and is a past trustee of the California Dental Association, and a member of the Board of Directors of the Northern California Society of Oral and Maxillofacial Surgeons. He is currently the secretary of the Osseointegration Foundation and the president of the Sadi Fontaine Academy. Bedrossian lectures extensively to his colleagues on treatment planning for oral surgical and implant patients. Bedrossian is a Diplomate of the American Board of Oral and Maxillofacial Surgeons and is a fellow of both the American College of Oral and Maxillofacial Surgeons and the American College of Dentists. He is a member of the American Dental

Association, the American Association of Oral and Maxillofacial Surgeons and the Pierre Fauchard Academy.

Bedrossian and his wife, Jasmine, live in San Francisco with their two children.

Dr. Bedrossian may be reached through www.sfimplants.com.

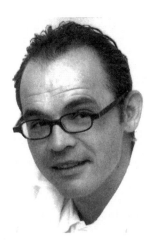

Peter S. Wöhrle, D.MD., M. Med.Sc., C.D.T., completed a four-year certified dental technician program (C.D.T.) in Switzerland. Subsequently, Wöhrle entered Harvard University, where he received his D.M.D. degree *cum laude* and was the recipient of the Norman B. Nesbett award for clinical excellence. Continuing his post-doctoral studies at Harvard, he completed the advanced education (specialty) program in prosthodontics followed by the advanced education program in implant dentistry. In addition, Wöhrle also holds a Masters of Medical Sciences degree in Oral Biology from Harvard.

Wöhrle has presented more than 100 lectures worldwide on the topic of implant dentistry. Some of his courses feature live surgeries, allowing colleagues to observe state-of-the-art procedures. Wöhrle has published more than thirty-five articles, book chapters, and abstracts in the professional literature, focusing on the development of new techniques to further improve patient care with dental implants. He is a pioneer in developing new treatment concepts in immediate loading of implants, both for full arches as well as for single teeth. Currently, Wöhrle is involved in developing a new, scalloped implant system that enhances esthetic outcome by minimizing bone remodeling.

He is a member of many professional organizations, including the Academy of Osseointegration and the American College of Prosthodontists.

Wöhrle's practice in Newport Beach, California, is limited to implant dentistry and prosthodontics; he provides a entire spectrum of implant treatments, both surgically and restoratively. He is one of the few dentists worldwide with formal training in the interrelated areas of implant surgery, implant prosthodontics, and implant laboratory technology.

Dr. Wöhrle may be reached through his Web Site: www.implantspecialist.com.

Other Consumer Health Titles from Addicus Books

Visit our online catalog at www.AddicusBooks.com

After Mastectomy—Healing Phsyically and Emotionally $14.95

Cancers of the Mouth and Throat A Patient's Guide to Treatment $14.95

Cataracts: A Patient's Guide to Treatment $14.95

Colon & Rectal Cancer—A Patient's Guide to Treatment $14.95

Coping with Psoriasis—A Patient's Guide to Treatment $14.95

Coronary Heart Disease—A Guide to Diagnosis and Treatment $15.95

Exercising Through Your Pregnancy $17.95

The Fertility Handbook—A Guide to Getting Pregnant $14.95

The Healing Touch—Keeping the Doctor/Patient Relationship
Alive Under Managed Care $9.95

The Macular Degeneration Source Book $14.95

LASIK—A Guide to Laser Vision Correction $14.95

Living with P.C.O.S.—Polycystic Ovarian Syndrome $14.95

Lung Cancer—A Guide to Treatment & Diagnosis $14.95

The Macular Degeneration Source Book $14.95

The Non-Surgical Facelift Book A Guide to Facial Rejuvenation Procedures $14.95

Overcoming Postpartum Depression and Anxiety. $14.95

A Patient's Guide to Dental Implants $14.95

Prescription Drug Addiction—The Hidden Epidemic $15.95

Simple Changes: The Boomer's Guide to a Healthier, Happier Life $9.95

A Simple Guide to Thyroid Disorders $14.95

Straight Talk About Breast Cancer $14.95

From Diagnosis to Recovery: The Stroke Recovery Book $14.95
 A Guide for Patients and Families

The Surgery Handbook—A Guide to Understanding Your Operation. . . . $14.95

Understanding Lumpectomy: A Treatment Guide for Breast Cancer $14.95

Understanding Parkinson's Disease: A Self-Help Guide $14.95

Organizatons, associations, corporations, hospitals, and other groups may qualify for special discounts when ordering more than 24 copies. For more information, please contact the Special Sales Department at Addicus Books. Phone (402) 330-7493. Email: info@AddicusBooks.com

Please send:

_____copies of _____
(Title of book)

at $_____each   TOTAL   _____

Nebr. residents add 5.5% sales tax   _____

Shipping/Handling
   $4.00 for first book.
   $1.00 for each additional book.   _____

   TOTAL ENCLOSED: _____

Name _____

Address _____

City_____State_____Zip _____

☐   Visa   ☐   Master Card   ☐   Am. Express

Credit card number _____Expiration date _____

Order by credit card, personal check or money order. Send to:

Addicus Books
Mail Order Dept.
P.O. Box 45327
Omaha, NE 68145
Or, order TOLL FREE: **800-352-2873**